THE ULTIMATE
SEX DIET

THE SECRET FORMULA

FOR A SLIMMER, HEALTHIER,

MORE PASSIONATE LIFE

THE ULTIMATE
SEX DIET

KERRY McCLOSKEY

BERKLEY BOOKS, NEW YORK

THE BERKLEY PUBLISHING GROUP
Published by the Penguin Group
Penguin Group (USA) Inc.
375 Hudson Street, New York, New York 10014, USA
Penguin Group (Canada), 90 Eglinton Avenue East, Suite 700, Toronto, Ontario M4P 2Y3, Canada
(a division of Pearson Penguin Canada Inc.)
Penguin Books Ltd., 80 Strand, London WC2R 0RL, England
Penguin Group Ireland, 25 St. Stephen's Green, Dublin 2, Ireland (a division of Penguin Books Ltd.)
Penguin Group (Australia), 250 Camberwell Road, Camberwell, Victoria 3124, Australia
(a division of Pearson Australia Group Pty. Ltd.)
Penguin Books India Pvt. Ltd., 11 Community Centre, Panchsheel Park, New Delhi—110 017, India
Penguin Group (NZ), Cnr. Airborne and Rosedale Roads, Albany, Auckland 1310, New Zealand
(a division of Pearson New Zealand Ltd.)
Penguin Books (South Africa) (Pty.) Ltd., 24 Sturdee Avenue, Rosebank, Johannesburg 2196,
South Africa

Penguin Books Ltd., Registered Offices: 80 Strand, London WC2R 0RL, England

PRINTING HISTORY
True Courage Press hardcover edition / October 2004
Berkley trade paperback edition / January 2007

Library of Congress Cataloging-in-Publication Data

McCloskey, Kerry.
  The Ultimate sex diet : the secret formula for a slimmer, healthier, more passionate life / Kerry
McCloskey.
    p. cm.
  ISBN-13: 978-0-425-21374-2
  1. Weight loss—Miscellanea.   2. Sex—Health aspects.   I. Title
RM222.2.M43345 2007
613.2'5—dc22   2006051671
PRINTED IN THE UNITED STATES OF AMERICA

10   9   8   7   6   5   4   3   2   1

Every effort has been made to ensure that the information contained in this book is complete
and accurate. However, neither the publisher nor the author is engaged in rendering professional advice or services to the individual reader. The ideas, procedures, and suggestions
contained in this book are not intended as a substitute for consulting with your physician. All
matters regarding your health require medical supervision. Neither the author nor the publisher shall be liable or responsible for any loss or damage allegedly arising from any information or suggestion in this book.

The publisher does not have any control over and does not assume any responsibility for author or third party websites or their content.

This book is warmly dedicated to my husband, Ben, and to my parents—thank goodness you all love sex!

CONTENTS

ACKNOWLEDGMENTS

My warmest thanks to my agent, Larry Kirshbaum, for his guidance and support. My thanks to Christine Zika and the staff at Berkley for believing in me. My thanks and appreciation to Toby Amid for working with me to perfect the Two-Week Sex Diet. I am also grateful to Milli Brown, Kathryn Grant, and Erica Jennings of Brown Books for their outstanding expert assistance in helping me to put this book together. My thanks to photographer Yoav Elkoby of YOMA Productions, New York, for taking the photographs that appear in this book, and to Andrew Simon for allowing me to further develop my comedic writing talents on www.doubleagent.com.

Thanks to my friends Misong Kim, Cara Hobbs, Natasha Lam, Kat Williams, Jiyeon Jeon, Matt Matzkin, Corrie Lyle, Brad Abelson, Eve Kriz, Shelley Liebsch, Nina Nho, Mike Gregorio, Rob Hospidor, and Alison Fragale, for their encouragement and positive influence on my life. Thanks also to "the future President," Damian (Scott) Dolyniuk, for instilling in me an optimistic point of view about the future. My appreciation to Nick Ragone for his advice and words of wisdom. My thanks to Jessica Hughes for giving me the idea and encouragement to write a book (though I know this one isn't what you had in mind).

My very special thanks to my parents for their insight, guidance, and creative inspiration. Thanks also to Nana for passing on the "sassy" genes and to my sisters, Allison and Rory, for their support, suggestions, love, loyalty, and friendship. Finally, an extra special thank you to my husband Ben for his love and help in "researching" the ideas used in the book.

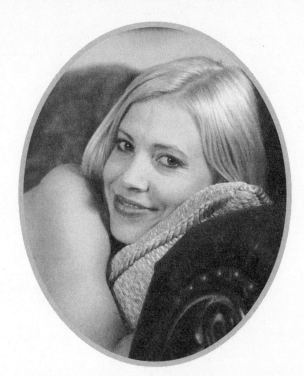

HOW I DISCOVERED THE ULTIMATE SEX DIET

have an amazing secret. It has changed my life. It has made me healthier and happier than ever before.

At work, my coworkers do not know my secret. Not even my family or closest friends realize the truth.

My secret has made my life so much richer, and so much more fun and exciting, that I cannot keep it bottled up inside of me any longer. I'm thrilled to share my discovery with you and I am confident it will change your life forever, too.

When I first started dating my husband, Ben, I was in the worst shape of my life. My stomach and buttocks were the flabbiest they had ever been, I rarely exercised, and every diet fad and gimmick I tried had led to failure and frustration. Luckily, my future husband was able to overlook my "flaws." In fact, by our third date we were head over heels in love and in the midst of a whirlwind romance that was filled with wonderfully long and satisfying lovemaking. Within the first three months of dating, I lost ten pounds without even trying. I had an uncanny feeling that my

I have an amazing secret. It has changed my life. It has made me healthier and happier than ever before.

boosted metabolism due to our intense sexual activity played a major role in helping me slim down.

However, when Ben and I settled into a more relaxed sexual routine, I stopped losing weight and eventually gained back five of the pounds I had lost. For the rest of our first year together, my weight stayed at a comfortable level, but as with many men and women, it was still twenty pounds above where I wanted it to be.

Within the first three months of dating, I lost ten pounds without even trying.

After Ben romantically proposed to me at the top of the Eiffel Tower on the anniversary of our first date, I rapidly began to lose weight again. My friends and family thought I was on a strict diet and exercise regimen for my wedding. The real truth was that Ben and I had once again unleashed our sexual desires and had become more sexually active than ever.

Other than doing a few toning exercises in the morning, I was not working out anywhere but the bedroom. Without even realizing it, I had also begun to eat healthier and had cut most of the sugar and the unhealthy types of carbs and fats out of my diet. I was only eating foods that made me feel good about myself and my health.

I suddenly realized that our high-energy sex life was the critical key to how great I felt and looked. It was a real-life example of cause and effect: The better I looked the more I wanted sex, and the more sex we had the better I looked. I was not thinking that logically, of course, but the results were the same nonetheless. "What about junk food?" you might ask. It was not until after I had binged on pizza and cookies

Bad eating habits affect your feelings about your body and yourself, and they hurt your sex drive.

one fateful day and was so exhausted that I denied Ben's advances that I had an epiphany: Foods that are bad for you make you feel even worse—not only physically, while you're digesting and absorbing them, but also emotionally. Bad eating habits affect your feelings about your body and yourself, and they hurt your sex drive. I witnessed the results of this "experiment" in my own bedroom. The junk food I had eaten made me lose interest in sex. I not only felt worse, but I also looked worse—and became even less interested in sex.

More cause and effect? I thought so.

Armed with this new knowledge, I continued my secret diet of eating healthier and having lots and lots of great sex. Amazingly, I lost a total of twenty-three pounds before my wedding.

Focusing on my problem areas during sex and contracting the right muscles at the right time also proved to be a great way to tone my body. Of course, I could not tell anyone about it at that point because I would have been admitting that I engaged in premarital sex. After all, Ben is Catholic and I was never even baptized! I was lucky they were even allowing a naughty girl like me to get married in a Catholic church.

Now that we've been happily married for more than four years, I can tell the world my secret. Since our marriage, I have not only kept the weight off, but I have done a tremendous amount of research on my accidental sex diet discovery and found that sex, in fact, provides enormous physical and psychological health benefits. It is also the easiest, most pleasurable way to lose weight.

> I continued my secret diet of eating healthier and having lots and lots of great sex. Amazingly, I lost a total of twenty-three pounds before my wedding.

Personally, I have not only lost a total of twenty-three pounds and kept them off, but I am also in a constant state of euphoria. I walk around surrounded by the happy glow that comes from all the love, sex, and intimacy Ben and I share on a regular basis. I can assure you that the glow is not just in my imagination; there is scientific evidence that sex is actually a "beauty treatment." Tests have found that when women make love, they produce more estrogen, which makes their hair shiny and smooth. Also, the sweat produced cleanses pores and makes the skin glow, reducing the chances of dermatitis and rashes. On top of this, my wonderful sex life has helped me build a healthy and satisfying marriage—both in and out of the bedroom—and I have never looked or felt better.

One last secret! For years before I met Ben, I had dreamed of becoming a model or an actress, but I had been rejected every time I tried out. Modeling agencies had no interest in me, nor was I given a second look at casting sessions. I was told every excuse in the book: You're too heavy, too old, too commercial-looking, and so on.

After I married Ben, I decided to give modeling one last shot. I knew the chances were slim, since at that point I was already twenty-seven years old, which was considered "ancient" by the ridiculous standards of the modeling industry (heck, I was "too old" since I was twenty-two)! However, I took the chance because I was finally feeling so good about myself.

So, knowing that I felt better than I ever had in my life, I had some photos taken of me and sent them to a few small agencies. EVERY ONE of them called me back! Obviously, I did not knock on the doors of the top ten New York modeling agencies, where it often seems that you have to be fifteen and anorexic to get a second look, but I did become a freelance model and began to get a steady stream of assignments through several small commercial agencies! I have not booked any modeling jobs that broke the bank, but for the past four years I have had consistent modeling work on television, starred in several fashion shows, appeared in several magazine layouts, and even worked as a leg model in a promotional ad for *Sex and the City*! Ben liked that one!

I should clarify that my modeling and acting jobs are only hobbies. I am a former high school valedictorian and National Merit Scholar. I graduated from an Ivy League college with a degree in Math and Economics. Also, as of February 2007, I will have a masters degree in health education from Columbia University. Currently, I work full-time as a director of marketing research for one of the largest media companies in the world. My career is challenging and very hectic, but I still make time for the important things in my life, such as my relationship with my husband. We make time to support each other, resolve our conflicts, and keep each other updated on everything in our lives, just as best friends should do. He is the number one priority in my life.

The funny thing is that when I look at pictures of myself when I was twenty-four, I realize that I looked older then than I do now at thirty-one! And it is not just me—researchers have found that ample sex helps you look between four to seven years younger because it helps you feel more content, sleep better, and feel less stressed. Hallelujah for sex . . . yes, yes, YES!

Surprisingly, the concept of this book is not new. There have been many studies and articles that have cited the health benefits of sex. You've probably read a few of them yourself. However, up until now, people have treated this information as nothing more than gossip, wishful thinking, or entertainment. We accept the general notion that sex is good for us in many ways, but we haven't really applied that critical information to our daily lives.

The idea that sex is healthy for us usually just results in a few laughs, or perhaps becomes an excuse to have some special fun that day, but no real lifestyle changes take place. Part of the problem is that many of these studies are quite vague on what you need to do to get all of the wonderful benefits of sex.

> **Researchers have found that ample sex helps you look between four to seven years younger because it helps you feel more content, sleep better, and feel less stressed.**

Though they touch on the subject of sex, they avoid the details of how and when to do the touching, arousing, and lovemaking. Most importantly, prior studies and articles have generally not emphasized the critical role that sex plays as an exercise that can help you slim down and shape up. This is the reason I decided to write this book.

Sex is no longer a taboo subject and even if it were, I am not afraid to talk about it. In fact, I will give you explicit directions on how to really make sex work for you. I will share with you the secrets I have gathered from my own personal experiences and the research I have done. I hope this information will change your life—and your sex life—forever.

I am excited to offer you a complete lifestyle program that has everything you need and want to know about sex as a tool to help you lose weight, improve your health, and be happier than ever. Obesity and depression continue to be national epidemics; this book has been written to help wipe them out!

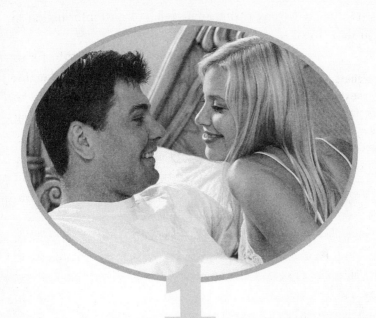

1

HAVE MORE FUN IN
BED . . . AND ON THE SCALE

Forget the Atkins diet. Celebrities have discovered a new way of staying in shape—and it's much more fun. The secret to a slimline figure is not cutting out carbs or saying no to chocolate, it's indulging in plenty of sex.

—*London Daily Mirror*, October 15, 2003

We have all heard the phrase "a healthy sexual appetite." Usually, it refers to an individual's ravenous desire for sex. However, after reading this book, you'll never look at this phrase the same way again. I will teach you how to increase your desire for sexual activity, help you lose weight, tone key areas, eat and feel healthier, and improve your overall attitude toward life, all through sex—the best workout program ever created, "patented" long ago by Adam and Eve!

Having sex feels great. If done right, we feel good during sex for the physical pleasure it provides, and we feel wonderful after sex for the emotional connection created through the romantic adventure with our partner. Many people, however, do not necessarily feel good about their bodies' appearance in general and especially not when they're making love. If this is the case, they cannot completely enjoy the experience.

> I will teach you how to increase your desire for sexual activity, help you lose weight, tone key areas, eat and feel healthier, and improve your overall attitude toward life, all through sex.

Like bears going into hibernation, some people dive beneath

the sheets as soon as they climax. It's certainly easy to lose the afterglow when a beam of light glimmers on the flab about which you're so self-conscious. People get so busy focusing on their rolls of unwanted fat that they forget all about the "meat"—the joy of giving and receiving love, which is, after all, the main ingredient in our human sandwich! This is a problem that plagues a large percentage of our population. In fact, studies have shown that the great majority of women think they're too fat. It's time to do something about that! To help you improve your body's shape and your body image is the primary reason I wrote this book. And what better way than with sex, on the Ultimate Sex Diet!

According to government studies by the Centers for Disease Control and Prevention, obesity plagues more than fifty-nine million Americans. Too many of us are overweight, overworked, and overwhelmed by life in general, and sex in particular. Too few of us find the time or the interest to get much exercise. I will elaborate on these concerns in Chapter 2, The Ultimate Exercise Machine, and in Chapter 3, Stress Relief: Undress to Decompress. The rest of the book will also provide guidance on how to address these problems.

I want everyone who reads this groundbreaking book to feel good about sex, to feel good during and after sex, and to use sex as a tool to improve their physical appearance and outlook on life. Of course, this primarily applies to adults who are involved in a monogamous relationship, or one in which safe sex is consistently practiced. The importance of having sex in a loving, monogamous relationship was hinted at by a Japanese study in which nineteen of forty-two people who had a stroke during sex were being unfaithful at the time. In a study entitled "Money, Sex, and Happiness," published by the National

Bureau of Economic Research in May 2004, Dartmouth College economist David Blanchflower and economist Andrew Oswald of Warwich University in England found that to maximize happiness, a person should have just one sexual partner. They discovered that "people who say they have ever paid for sex are considerably less happy than others. Those who have ever had sex outside their marriage also report notably low happiness."

Just as too much exercise, or the wrong kind of exercise, can be counterproductive, not all sexual activity falls within the realm of the Ultimate Sex Diet. For instance, scientific studies show that having sex with multiple partners can increase a man's risk of getting cancer or certain other diseases by up to 40 percent. That's because he runs a greater risk of contracting a sexually related infection that might compromise his immune system.

Moreover, certain relationships give you a head start toward getting the most benefit from making love. For example, if you marry your partner, you are more likely to engage in sex more frequently. According to a 1998 study performed at the University of Chicago, married couples engage in sexual activity 25–300 percent more often than nonmarried people, depending on age.

On top of that, decades of research has clearly shown that marriage increases your life span. Over twice as many divorced and widowed men, and one and a half times as many single men, die before married men do. This expanded life span also applies to married women. About 10 percent more wives outlive single women, and 50 percent more outlive divorcees and widows. Apparently, "happily ever after" really means happily ever after—plus a few more years.

Sex helps you live longer, whether the positive benefits stem from your body or your mind.

A study at Duke University that followed 270 men and women over a span of twenty-five years reinforced these findings. It determined that "frequency of intercourse was a significant predictor of longevity for men while enjoyment of intercourse was a predictor for women." So it seems that sex helps you live longer, whether the positive benefits stem from your body or your mind.

Living in America, we are raised to hide our bodies' flaws whenever possible. This is something that should apply only when you are out in public, and not in the privacy of your bedroom with your committed lover. Your partner should love you regardless of the shape your body is in.

Often, your partner does love you for better or for worse, so you alone hurt your self-image when you complain about your least favorite body parts and do nothing to change them.

Many women use the images of supermodels in bikinis, whom they see on television or in magazines, to give them the incentive to lose weight. Unfortunately, this practically ensures failure since most women lack the body type to ever look like these supermodels. Instead of helping you lose weight, these images can actually make you feel inferior, leading to depression and binge eating.

I will teach you to use a more effective incentive to slim down by using your imagination and focusing on you. The imagery in your mind of a more sensual you is a much more realistic and tangible motivational tool than some airbrushed, touched-up photo from a glossy fashion magazine. In Chapter 4, Body Image: Feeling Hot, Hot, HOT, I'll show you how to boost your self-confidence and perception of yourself.

Many people lose weight at the start of a new relationship. The excitement of a new love can temporarily speed up their metabolism. The constant thinking about food when you're single is replaced with loving thoughts of the new special person in your life. New lovers may also feel motivated to improve their appearance to further attract the ones they love, with the hope that the object of their affection will reciprocate their love. When the "honeymoon period" ends, however, the pounds often quickly return. Couples eventually reach a level of comfort with each other and spend more and more of their time together socializing while eating and drinking. They begin to feel more secure and often "let themselves go." This is when being part of a couple can negatively influence eating habits, particularly when one partner is less health-conscious than the other. The bad habits of each partner inevitably begin to transfer to the other.

Then it's the Ultimate Sex Diet to the rescue! It will motivate both of you to maintain a constant, intense level of frequent and pleasurable sexual activity.

That is why the Ultimate Sex Diet is most effective when both partners participate. It is still effective (and beneficial for both parties) with just one of you on the diet, but ideally both partners should be involved so that a positive transference prevails over a negative one.

Speaking of downers, the word "diet" can have a negative connotation. It is not a coincidence that the first three letters of the word spell "die." Most of us feel like we want to die when we are limiting our food intake. So, instead of viewing this as a "Sex Diet," I personally choose to replace the "i" with a "u" (coincidentally, a great strategy in

This diet is not about restrictions and deprivation. It is about celebrating, feeling, and indulging in life.

the bedroom), and view the Ultimate Sex Diet as a "Sex Duet Exercise and Nutritional Program," to give it a more positive ring.

I think a sex duet sounds fun, and indeed it is! This is also an appropriate term to use for our particular purposes, since sex involves two parties "singing" together, instead of just one person doing a solo. The most positive outcome of this interactive slimming program is that your partnership ultimately benefits just as much as each of you do. In Chapter 5, Feeling Sexy Every Night, you'll learn how both you and your partner can work together to achieve your unique diet goals.

The first step of the Ultimate Sex Diet is to make your whole food experience more sensual. The key is not only to focus on healthier foods that make you feel good while eating them, but also to fully appreciate the entire sensation of eating. You will soon discover that this diet is not about restrictions and deprivation. It is about celebrating, feeling, and indulging in life.

When food and eating are associated with the benefits derived from more intense foreplay, sex, and afterglow, your entire approach to food changes for the better.

"How can that be?" you might be wondering. Just think about how many negative attitudes you have about food. Traditional diets do nothing but reinforce these "bad food vibes." But when food and eating are associated with the benefits derived from more intense foreplay, sex, and afterglow, your entire approach to food changes for the better.

Like many areas of our lives, when it comes to eating and making love we need to take more time to completely enjoy what we experience. You need to enjoy the scent, the texture, the taste, and the feelings that are created when you eat, just as when you are making love. On the Ultimate Sex Diet you will be encouraged to try new exotic and sensual foods. Won't that be fun?!

In Chapter 12, Sexual Nutrition: Healthy Foods for Healthy

Loving, I will discuss how to approach food in a way that will heighten your sensory experience and how to translate these techniques into the bedroom. I will also discuss foods that are sexy to eat, those that serve as aphrodisiacs, and foods that can actually be used in the bedroom to enhance your sexual experiences.

In Chapter 14, Fighting Cravings: Don't Crave Sweets, Crave Your Sweetie, I will teach you how to fight your food cravings. You will learn how to transform a craving for junk food into a craving for your partner. (Move over Baby Ruth—I'm looking for Mr. Goodbar!) Many times we eat when we are not hungry, to fill an emotional void. I will tell you why that void exists in the first place and discuss the body movements, mind tricks, and various mental strategies specifically designed to fill the void without filling your belly!

> The tantalizing question becomes, are we dieting to have more sex, or are we having more sex to diet?

If you've been watching the news lately, you may have heard that there are many health benefits associated with sex. These include longer life spans, better cardiovascular health (surprise! sex really helps the heart), higher pain tolerances, an improved immune system, and a lower rate of depression. Chapter 16, Sexual Healing: The Amazing Health Benefits of Sex, will detail what science has discovered about the dramatic and positive impact sex can have on your physical well-being.

Now the tantalizing question becomes, are we dieting to have more sex, or are we having sex to diet? You will love the chapters devoted to what some have fondly called "Sexercise." This is an activity many of us have been engaging in for years without realizing the benefits we were reaping. Such lack of awareness caused us to miss opportunities to increase those benefits. If you've ever had sore muscles the morning after a good night of lovemaking, you may have been sexercising without even realizing it.

Aerobically, a half-hour romp in the sheets burns approximately 150–250 calories and sometimes even 350 calories if you are frisky enough. This is roughly the equivalent of briskly walking, running, or lifting weights for thirty minutes. Now which would you rather do: make sensual love with a warm partner, or just have a sweaty session on a cold and clammy exercise machine? The regular calorie "burning" from sex doesn't even include the additional calories used up during the strength and toning exercises you will learn about in Chapters 7, 8, and 9. Using my tantalizing suggestions for increasing the amount of foreplay involved in sex will burn up even more calories and also increase the amount of time you spend making love. These exercises will not only improve your body's appearance, they will also enhance your pleasure during sex and lead to greater orgasms. You'll be thanking me sooner than you think!

As you will discover, sex is a great exercise, and the more exercise you do in general, the better your sex life will be. Researchers at the University of California at San Diego found that three to four one-hour workouts per week helped men achieve steadier, more satisfying sex sessions with their partners. In a Harvard School of Public

> Aerobically, a half-hour romp in the sheets burns approximately 150–250 calories and sometimes even 350 calories if you are really frisky.

> The more you exercise, the more sex you have, and the more sex you have, the more exercise you are getting! Isn't this the most natural and most pleasurable way to really lose weight and keep it off?

Health study, men who worked out vigorously for twenty to thirty minutes several times a week reduced their risk of erection problems by half. Researchers at the University of Texas at Austin discovered that women's genital blood flow after watching an X-rated film was much greater after exercising than it was without the workout.

So, it's an amazing cycle: The more you exercise, the more sex you have, and the more sex you have, the more exercise you are getting! Isn't this the most natural and most pleasurable way to really lose weight and keep it off? Isn't this one of the best ways to get healthier and happier? Isn't life great? Yes!

2

THE ULTIMATE EXERCISE MACHINE

What was the steamy secret to Academy Award–winning actress Angelina Jolie's fabulous figure in her 2001 movie *Tomb Raider*? Although she worked out with weights, she revealed to Britain's *NOW* magazine that she wasn't just pumping iron. Frequent, passionate sex did the trick: "Having sex with my husband keeps me in much more shape."

—*Salon*, January 29, 2001

Why do you need to go on the Ultimate Sex Diet? Of course, your key motivations are to get slimmer, look better than ever, and have the most satisfying lovemaking of your life. However, there may be another really important reason you need to go on this diet. Look at your body in the mirror. Are you overweight? If not, are you concerned about becoming overweight in the future? If you answered yes to either of these questions, you're not alone.

The Obesity Epidemic

According to the National Health and Nutrition Examination surveys, over 65 percent of Americans are overweight. Nearly 25 percent of the population is "obese," a term referring to those at least thirty pounds over their recommended weight. Sadly, the obesity epidemic is getting worse. Twenty years ago, less than half of America's population was overweight. Today, Americans are ten pounds heavier on average than we were ten years ago. But obesity is not just an American problem. Nearly one-fourth of the world's population is overweight. The number of obese Britons has more than doubled since 1980. More than

50 percent of adults in the European Union are overweight or obese. In China, obesity increased ninefold just during the 1990s. A World Health Organization study noted that, while hunger and infectious diseases remain important problems, obesity will soon surpass them as the most severe public health problem facing the world.

Health experts generally agree on the causes of the obesity epidemic: our poor eating habits and our lack of exercise. We eat too many of the wrong foods, our portions are too large, and we are too physically inactive.

In a 2004 health study involving 4,700 adults, it was discovered that, despite the enormous number of books on low-carbohydrate, low-fat, fruit, and exotic diets that we are constantly buying, soft drinks and pastries still make up the greatest percentage of the calories we consume on a daily basis. The head of the study, Gladys Block, a professor of epidemiology and public health nutrition at the University of California at Berkeley, remarked that the most alarming part of the study was the prominent role that empty calories (foods with very little nutritional content) still play in the American diet. *The study found that sweets, desserts, soda, and alcohol account for nearly 25 percent of all calories consumed by Americans.* These are empty calories that do not contribute meaningful amounts of nutrients or vitamins to the body. In fact, your body can be undernourished while you are indulging in these non-nutritious foods. Block remarked that "[W]e know people are eating a lot of junk food, but to have almost one-third of Americans' calories coming from those cate-

There are countless health implications that go along with being overweight. Not only can it increase your blood pressure, it also puts you at risk for such diseases as cancer, diabetes, and arthritis, and can even dramatically reduce your life span.

gories is a shocker. It's no wonder there's an obesity epidemic in this country." Don't these people realize the prominent role of jelly rolls in creating body rolls? Wouldn't they rather roll in bed?

There are countless health implications that go along with being overweight. Not only can it increase your blood pressure, it also puts you at risk for such diseases as cancer, diabetes. and arthritis, and can even dramatically reduce your life span. Obesity is increasingly becoming recognized as a fatal epidemic; only smoking has a greater damaging impact. Researchers for the Journal of the American Medical Association found that very obese Caucasian persons have reduced their life spans by eight to thirteen years.

Recent findings indicate that the harmful results of being obese come not just from the stress of carrying around the extra weight, but also from the actual fat cells contained in the flesh of heavier people. According to Dr. Rudolph Leibel of Columbia University, "[W]hen we look at fat tissue now, we see it's not just a passive depot of fat, [but that] it's an active manufacturer of signals to other parts of the body." New scientific studies suggest that all fat storage cells create a mixture of hormones and other chemical messengers that affect the body's energy balance. When these cells are expanded with fat, they have a dangerous impact on many of the body's organs. Precisely how this happens is still being researched. However, scientists believe unequivocally that the biological consequences of being overweight may hasten death from heart disease, stroke, diabetes, and cancer.

Another hazard associated with enlarged fat cells is their effect on the body's production and usage of insulin, the hormone that regulates how muscles burn energy and how much is stored in fat cells. Scientists have found that elevated insulin levels can directly harm the walls of arteries and cause them to clog.

According to Dr. Michael Thun, chief of epidemiology at the American Cancer Society, "[T]here is now conclusive evidence that obesity causes some cancers and strong evidence that it contributes to a wide variety of others." The American Cancer Society estimates that staying fit could eliminate 90,000 cancer deaths in the United States each year. The cancers that have been most clearly linked to excess weight are cancers of the breast, uterus, colon, kidney, esophagus, pancreas, and gallbladder.

> Exercise strengthens the heart, improves respiratory capacity, builds energy, lowers blood pressure, improves muscle strength and tone, strengthens bones, reduces body fat and weight, and reduces the risk of certain diseases and medical conditions.

On top of all of its other health problems, being overweight may also decrease your sex drive! Those who are overweight often have less desire for sex because they may feel insecure about their body and sexually unattractive. Such insecurity could make them more susceptible to depression. I'd be depressed too if I had less desire for sex!

Our Lack of Exercise

It's a shame more Americans do not exercise. Studies show that exercise strengthens the heart, improves respiratory capacity, builds energy, lowers blood pressure, improves muscle tone and strength, strengthens bones, reduces body fat and weight, and reduces the risk of certain diseases and medical conditions such as type 2 diabetes and high blood pressure.

Does this mean that you need to run a marathon every week or climb Mount Everest to get in shape? No, not at all. Many researchers have found that even moderate exercise is highly beneficial to our health. A study by Danish experts completed in 2000 showed that any kind of exercise, even moderate exercise, could increase our life spans. Other studies have shown that even the most inactive people could gain significant health benefits by thirty minutes or more of physical activity per day. Experts recommend that each of us engage in twenty to thirty minutes of moderate-intensity aerobic exercise, such as walking, three times per week. They also encourage moderate anaerobic exercise, such as muscle strengthening and stretching activities, twice per week. It is suggested that, if you've been physically inactive for a while, you should start exercising again at a slow, comfortable pace so you can increase your fitness without straining yourself.

> **Many researchers have found that even moderate exercise is highly beneficial to our health.**

A 2003 study headed by John Jakicic, Ph.D., the director of the Physical Activity and Weight Management Research Center at the University of Pittsburgh, discovered that overweight women who combined dieting with moderate workouts lost nearly as much weight as those on intense exercise programs. According to Dr. Jakicic, ". . . it appears that intensity is not the main factor impacting long-term weight loss," but rather, consistency. Doing some regular exercise on a regular basis, "even accumulated in bouts of as little as ten minutes at a time," was the key to taking off the excess pounds and keeping them off.

The key to the best personal exercise programs, according to many physical fitness experts, is to find an activity you enjoy and have fun doing.

Unfortunately, most Americans have not changed their lifestyles to become more active. What is their solution? To buy more exercise equipment. To buy more memberships to

> **The key to the best personal exercise programs is to find an activity you enjoy and have fun doing.**

gyms. But beyond the limited exercise afforded by carrying the exercise equipment to its "final resting place" in the closet or in the basement, and the three or four visits to the gym before we get too "busy" to show up again, these purchases rarely result in successful efforts to meaningfully reduce our weight and get the exercise we need.

Perhaps one of the most overlooked ways to get fit and trim does not involve buying exercise equipment or buying gym club memberships. In fact, it does not involve buying anything. It's free. What is it? We are going to discover that one of the best exercise regimens ever created starts with you in your birthday suit. Without any exercise clothes (or any other clothes on). And with your partner in his or her birthday suit. Get the two of you fooling around and having fun in your birthday suits together more often and more vigorously, and you will have the best birthday (suit) parties—the kind that will help you enjoy many more actual birthdays with each other.

Being overweight or obese is a chronic condition and there are several contributing factors. A combination of genes, metabolism, behavior, environment, cultural influences, and socioeconomic status help determine an individual's body weight and shape. Obviously, dieting and exercise cannot change your gene pool, cultural influences, or socioeconomic status. However, the remaining three factors—metabolism, behavior, and environment—can all be addressed and altered by following the right program. Attention to nutrition and regular physical activity can reduce obesity, and may reduce such health risks as heart disease, diabetes, and osteoporosis.

Metabolism, behavior, and environment can also be influenced by an individual's life choices. If a choice is made to commit to the Ultimate Sex Diet, this program will impact all three factors and your weight could be dramatically reduced. Your metabolism will be influenced if the types of calories you consume are healthier for your digestive system; it will be further influenced by the exercises and sexercises that become part of your life. Behavior and environment will also change because I will arm you with the tools necessary to reduce stress, feel better about yourself, and have a better relationship with your partner.

Even if a couple's relationship is so great it would rate a "10" on a scale of 1 to 10, it is discouraging when the couple also looks like the number 10 when standing next to each other. Additionally, excess size and weight place physical limitations on the types of sexual positions that can be enjoyed when fooling around in the bedroom.

Get the two of you fooling around and having fun in your birthday suits together more often and more vigorously, and you will have the best birthday (suit) parties—the kind that will help you enjoy many more actual birthdays with each other.

Therefore, the Ultimate Sex Diet will be more than a diet and exercise program for you. This is a lifestyle makeover. The differences will be apparent in every aspect of your life, including your interactions with others. You'll love to begin looking in the mirror, at your body and at your partner's body, more and more often. Ultimately, the most important change will be the transition from one big "O" (obesity) to a slimmer physique and a better "O" (orgasm)!

Therefore, the Ultimate Sex Diet will be more than a diet and exercise program for you. This is a lifestyle makeover.

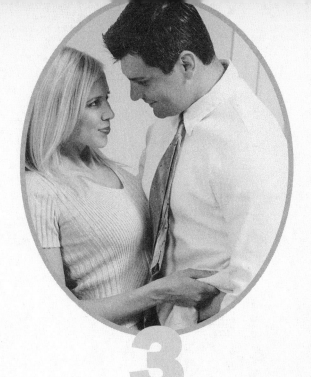

3

STRESS RELIEF:
UNDRESS TO DECOMPRESS

"Sex can be a very effective way of reducing stress levels," says clinical psychologist Karen Donahey, Ph.D., director of the Sex and Marital Therapy Program at Northwestern University Medical Center. "Having sex chills a guy out, suffuses him with a profound feeling of well-being and relaxation. . . . [I]t's much easier to be optimistic if there's a chance that at any moment your wife might pull you into the hall closet and give you a good going-over."

—Hugh O'Neill and Tom McGrath, *Men's Health*, November 1997

W hat is it that often keeps you from making love as often as you and your partner would like? S-T-R-E-S-S. As DiscoveryHealth.com noted on April 19, 2004, "All too often . . . we haven't the time or energy for sex. According to the Masters & Johnson Institute, at least a third of American couples experience a lack of desire. After a stressful day at work [or at home!] it's easy to neglect the ultimate celebration of human pleasure."

> When the sad, sorry spirits of stress come knocking at your door, who are you going to call? How are you going to spell relief? You guessed it . . . S-E-X!

When the sad, sorry spirits of stress come knocking at your door, who are you going to call? How are you going to spell relief? You guessed it . . . S-E-X! It's one of those ridiculous cycles: You're too stressed for sex, yet sex has been proven to relieve stress. This is similar to other ironies that we'll mention later, such as you don't want sex because you have a headache, yet sex can help relieve headaches. Around and around we

> Sex can change your attitude and relax you, giving you a better perspective on how to deal with the chaos of life.

go. *It's time to stop going around and around and instead to start going up and down!*

Stress is an important ailment to address. Scientific evidence suggests that stress can exacerbate existing illnesses; it can also increase the odds of experiencing other health problems including chronic fatigue, heart attacks, and autoimmune diseases such as lupus and rheumatoid arthritis. Atlanta psychologist Robert Simmermon, Ph.D., has found that stress can also be contagious, spreading rapidly among those in contact with a stressed-out individual. This is especially true within families.

Now, I know making love more often won't change your hectic schedule or the fact that you may have work, kids, chores, finances, and errands to juggle all at once. Sex can, however, change your attitude and relax you, giving you a better perspective on how to deal with the chaos of life. All work and no play makes for a dull and frustrating life in more ways than one. You may feel so pressured that you make little time to make love. Remember, there is always time for sex. A half-hour of television can be sacrificed for a half-hour of fun in the sheets. You'll actually feel more relaxed and mellow.

I also strongly encourage you to make sex dates. Less spontaneity in exchange for much more frequent sexual activity is a "sacrifice" you should be very willing to make. In fact, having a sex date can actually increase anticipation and make the loving more thrilling. Alternate who plans the foreplay activity and who chooses the sex position. Build your partner's curiosity and do a little teasing during the hours leading up to the lovemaking. That builds the intensity of the activity and revitalizes your sex drive. Your passion will feel as hot as it was at the beginning of your relationship, when you first wanted to make love with your partner and immediately felt the desire to jump into bed together.

The ensuing feelings of satisfaction and relaxation can do wonders for your emotional state and simultaneously reduce your stress. Dennis Foley, author of *As Good As It Gets*, cites a recent study indicating that sex serves as a sedative and reduces anxiety and stress. In fact, even fantasizing about sex can be calming and has been shown to reduce depression and anger.

According to Bryant Stamford, Ph.D., professor and director of the health promotion center at the University of Louisville, sex does not get enough respect for its tension-relieving qualities. He explained in WebMD on January 23, 2004, that "sex and love are the Rodney Dangerfield of stress management." He added that because of all the negative energy we take in during the day, the stress-relieving impact of sex is a very positive benefit.

Sex is also exercise and is, therefore, the ideal stress reliever.

Exercise is also a great remedy for stress. According to Tim McCall, writing in a 2001 *Redbook* magazine article, exercise works on several levels, triggering physical changes that boost your fitness and self-esteem. As discussed in the prior chapter, regular exercise improves the function of your immune system. In addition, it prevents your mental ability from drastically declining with age. Sex is also exercise and is, therefore, the ideal stress reliever. If you feel too stressed for sex, I'm confident that sex will make you feel less stressed.

4

BODY IMAGE:
FEELING HOT, HOT, HOT

Anyone who has been swept off his or her feet knows that romance can do wonders for the waistline. The thrill of the unknown, the butterflies in the stomach, and the head-in-the-clouds forgetfulness all ensure that overeating is not on the agenda. And that's before the physical demands of all the steamy sex make the weight drop off. A half-hour session can burn up to 350 calories—the same as a 30-minute run.

—*London Daily Mirror*, October 15, 2003

Does your view of how you look hurt your desire for sex? Are you afraid that your body image—and your body—are turning off your spouse? In fact, do you ever have days when you think you look like a big fat box of glazed donuts? Do you then feed your depression with the very evil that got you there in the first place? Are you then so upset about the half dozen donuts in your belly that you sit around the house moping, knowing that a gym visit would be pointless

Next time skip the donuts, the ice cream, and the potato chips and head straight back to bed.

since it would take a full five hours of boring, painful running just to burn off the 2,000 calories you've just consumed? Well, stop being depressed! Next time skip the donuts, the ice cream, and the potato chips and head straight back to bed. But not alone. That's right! Learn how much more comforting making wild love with your partner is than gorging on the "comfort foods" that are destroying your body, your love life, and your self-confidence. And keep on nibbling on your partner until you're full. NO, DON'T TAKE BITES OF EACH OTHER. I WAS JUST KIDDING! It's important to maintain a good sense of humor at all times, especially when you're trying to lose weight.

First of all, why would anyone ever eat donuts? Can't they see that the word "donut" is one letter away from spelling "do not"? Yes, they taste good, but the hole in the middle doesn't mean that the empty space is saving calories or fat. If you had a glob of carbs, sugar, and fat and put a hole in the middle, it would still be a glob of carbs, sugar, and fat—which is exactly what a donut is.

Now, on a more serious note, here's how to change your negative feelings about yourself. To start, open your closet. Identify any articles of clothing that make you look heavier than you actually are and set them aside permanently; better yet, give them to Goodwill. Too many people own clothing that they hate, that is not flattering, and that may cause a stomach or rear end to appear larger than it really is. This is simply poor planning.

Don't wait until you reach your ideal weight to buy the clothes that look good on you and make you look trim. Even if you weigh more than you would like, you can't get motivated to lose weight if you look terrible on a daily basis. Looking terrible leads to feeling terrible, and it's just plain inconsiderate to your partner. Besides, buying some new clothes before you lose weight will increase your incentive to continue dropping the pounds. There's no better feeling in the world than trying on a pair of pants that used to look fabulous on you, and now they look atrocious—because they're too big!

> There's no better feeling in the world than trying on a pair of pants that used to look fabulous on you, and now they look atrocious—because they're too big!

Keep "sexy" in mind when you go shopping. Of course, this does not mean you have to buy clothes that make you look like a "street girl." Buy tasteful clothes that make you feel and look desirable. Buy colors that complement you, and pay close attention to texture. Silk is sensual; polyester may not be. Cheaper fabrics can also make you sweat more, and body odor is not appealing. Clothing that feels good on you and makes you look good is not just wonderful for you; your partner will also enjoy touching it—and removing it!

Buy tasteful clothes that make you feel and look desirable.

Ladies, that goes double for undergarments. Of course, comfort is most important, but does it really boost your self-confidence when you know that under your clothes you're wearing raggedy underwear or "granny panties"? Also, wear matching bras and panties. It just makes you look and feel sexier. Even if you don't have all matching sets, at least color coordinate. This advice goes for men, too. Your underwear can't double as a girdle. Wearing a pair of underwear that results in belly overhang and leaves a red irritated elastic mark on your stomach will not improve your self-image or your love life.

The most important fashion item a woman can own is sexy shoes. Yes, comfort is important, but high heels are great for working out the calves and they make your legs look much sleeker and longer. On top of that, they just make you feel more desirable. Do you feel better about yourself when you're in a sleek, strappy pair of stilettos or slides, or when you're in an old beat-up pair of clunkers? Shoes are also important for men. You want to look like a cool guy, not like a homeless person, so wear stylish shoes that are in good condition.

Finally, grooming is important. Maintain a hairstyle that makes you look youthful and sexy. Keep your fingernails clean and trim. Make sure your teeth are white and brushed. Shave or wax off unsightly body hair. Most importantly, keep clean, very clean. Except in bed, of course, where it's okay to get a little dirty sometimes. Make sure you use an effective deodorant and even some fragrant soap, shower gel, and (on the right occasions) perfume or cologne. Don't forget to keep your skin moisturized so that it looks supple and inviting. Dry skin is not appealing, especially when it's a-peeling!

As often as possible, make the effort to look as if you were going out on a first date. Remember all the effort you made to look attractive and sexy before going out with your partner for the first time? That's where all the passion started. To continue the joys and pleasures of staying together, you need to continue to seduce each other and exude the confidence and chemistry that was there at the outset of the relationship. These are the juices that initially got your mutual passions raging. Of course, you don't have to look like Hollywood stars who just spent hours with makeup artists to feel good about yourselves and stay attracted to each other. Remember, your lover adores you and is turned on by you because you are you—a wonderful person, and not just a "celebrity face." You do, however, need to make a continuing effort to make yourself attractive and sexy to your partner.

We have discussed the first steps to improving your body image, which should put you in the right frame of mind to abstain from binging mindlessly on fatty, starchy, or sugary foods because you feel bad about your body. Now, let's dig a little deeper into your psyche. Self-esteem is not

> Most importantly, keep clean, very clean. Except in bed, of course, where it's okay to get a little dirty sometimes.

> To continue the joys and pleasures of staying together, you need to continue to seduce each other and exude the confidence and chemistry that was there at the outset of the relationship.

what other people think of you; it's what you think of yourself, so only you can change it. Only you can control your own thoughts. The power of your own words cannot be underestimated. Your first step every morning should be to stand naked in front of a mirror and repeat this mantra: "I am damn sexy! I have amazing (insert your favorite body parts). I look good, I am great in bed, and I reek of sex appeal. I am a rock star in the bedroom." Add any phrases that you find particularly sexy and gratifying. A large part of your motivation to do anything, including losing weight and increasing your sexual enjoyment, is your mental state. If your mental state is a positive one, your body will become ready, willing, and able to give and receive pleasure!

Now, there will be times when that negative inner voice will enter your mind and wage an internal war against you. Your strategy will be to be prepared for combat. As soon the negative voice appears and tries to make you feel bad about yourself, be ready to fight it with a vengeance. When it whispers about beautiful anorexic models, or about how large your thighs are, confront it immediately before the negativity overwhelms you. Recognize that even your own brain is capable of attacking your self-confidence and best intentions. Keep the security alert on at all times. When you hear the discouraging inner voice approaching, raise the alert to Code Red and be ready to destroy it with the knowledge of your great qualities and features, of the people who love you for yourself, of the progress you've already made to meet your personal goals, and of your determination to look and be your best. Take that, you evil little voice! POW!

Your body image is, of course, most important when you are

> If your mental state is a positive one, your body will become ready, willing, and able to give and receive pleasure!

in your most vulnerable position—naked in the bedroom. The Fox TV show *Arrested Development* had a character with a psychological problem known as a "Never Nude." He always left at least a pair of jean shorts on because he dreaded being naked. On a certain level, I am sure many of us can relate to the feeling of wanting to be a "Never Nude."

A recent *Psychology Today* survey indicated that 56 percent of women are dissatisfied with their bodies. Their biggest concerns are their abdomens (71 percent), their weight (66 percent), their hips (61 percent), and their muscle tone (57 percent). So it is time that we all faced the naked truth: None of us has a perfect body! We all need to get over our "faults" and onto our partners.

> So it is time that we all faced the naked truth: None of us has a perfect body!

Getting comfortable while being naked starts with getting to know yourself in the mirror. Remember the morning mantra we discussed above; repeat it throughout the day (though not too loudly in public!). Stand naked in front of the mirror as often as possible. Get to know your body's flaws and imperfections, and accept the ones you cannot change. Do not be afraid of these "flaws," because the more familiar you are with them, the more comfortable you will be. Then, as you shed the pounds on this sexy diet and exercise program, you will begin to see improvements in how you look and feel and it will give you the motivation and confidence to keep on playin' and shapin'. Always keep in mind that while the flaws are the parts of your body you focus on most, your partner does not, just as you don't focus on his. In fact, CNN reported on August 16, 1999, that men are more turned on by women's responsiveness in bed than they are by any particular body part.

When you're looking in the mirror, also be sure to focus on the many great-looking parts of your body. Glance at your anatomy and appreciate the incredible wonder of the human body. Allow your imagination to wander; visualize what you want your body to look like

> Remember, it is the way you think about yourself and carry yourself that makes you sexy.

and the further sensual adventures that await you on the Ultimate Sex Diet. Remember, it is the way you think about yourself and carry yourself that makes you sexy.

A problem many of us share is that we often take our insecurities out on our partners. No bed, home, or relationship is big enough for these hurtful actions. We need to quash the negative thoughts and stop blaming others. As Eleanor Roosevelt said, "No one can make you feel inferior without your permission." When your partner adoringly pats your belly, it doesn't mean that you are fat! When your partner squeezes your rear end as you walk by, it is a gesture of love, not a hint to firm the flab (unless, of course, they are misguided people whose negativity must be rechanneled into more

> Always discuss and praise each other's best features and strengthen each other's confidence, self-image, and self-worth.

considerate behavior!). We also need to be better about praising our partners. We need to consider which of their features and characteristics makes them feel really good about themselves. Heap on the compliments before, during, and after sex, and you will both be rewarded with the outcome. Be sure the compliments you give are 100 percent genuine and sincere. Always discuss and praise each other's best features and strengthen each other's confidence, self-image, and self-worth. Work hard to keep each other in the most positive frames of mind. It will keep you truly happy, and not just inside your bedroom.

Make sure to indulge in the whole sexual experience and appreciate every part of it. Take your time in the moments leading up to sex. Slowly remove your clothing and your partner's. You may even enjoy doing a little striptease to build up the excitement. You'll feel sexy while being playful and both of you will have fun. Music can also enhance the sexual experience. If a song is playing that makes you feel sexy and turns you on, it will help focus your attention away from any remaining insecurities about your body.

Your body confidence also impacts how you feel during sex. Your sexual experience is so much better when you're both feeling good about yourselves and you focus on the physical feelings of pleasure rather than on your internal doubts, problems, and insecurities. Focus on the sensation of flesh against flesh; on the intense tingling in your lips, breasts, arms, and legs; and on the concentrated erotic enjoyment you are feeling in the most intimate parts of your body. Your partner will be more turned on when you exude confidence and let go of your inhibitions in the bedroom. If you have a particular feature you are still insecure about, find a position that is the most flattering angle for it. If you are most insecure about your rear end, climb on top and face your partner. If your stomach is your biggest insecurity, stay on the bottom; your stomach will appear to be flatter and won't jiggle as much. In Chapters 8 and 9, we will get into the specifics of how to actually tone these areas during foreplay and while you're making love.

Just remember, if you don't allow your insecurities to enter your bedroom with you, then each night the two of you will be wonderfully alone to enjoy, enjoy, enjoy . . .

> Just remember, if you don't allow your insecurities to enter the bedroom with you, then each night the two of you will be wonderfully alone to enjoy, enjoy, enjoy . . .

5

FEELING SEXY EVERY NIGHT

Around 43 percent of women and 31 percent of men are sexually dysfunctional . . . The leading culprit seems to be a lack of libido—a general disinterest in sex . . . And how important, really, is a hot sex life in a committed relationship? Very important, indeed! It has been found that couples enjoying great sex report a higher quality of life. They experience less depression. Regular intimacy is the perfect buffer for the stress in our lives—helping us to stay healthy and happy.

—Deb Donovan and Bob VanMetter, IVillage.com

The fun of the Ultimate Sex Diet is that you can do it as a couple, as a "Sex Duet." We all know how difficult it can be when one partner is trying to diet and is grumpy all the time, while the other partner indulges in hamburgers and French fries. It just does not feel fair and can become a source of strife in the relationship. It is also frustrating if one person is on a diet and feels like they are making great strides with their body's appearance and the other person does not even notice. You do not want to fish for a compliment, but many of us rely on our partners to make us feel better about ourselves and reinforce our efforts. On the Ultimate Sex Diet, each partner is required to notice and compliment the other on the hard work and progress being made.

The fun of the Ultimate Sex Diet is that you can do it as a couple, as a "Sex Duet."

The key to this diet is that it won't feel like you're both suffering together. Instead, you will both be having fun together, and indulging in each other. The best part of all is that both of you will look better and also feel closer. Between looking at each other, and looking at yourselves, your hormones will be raging like you were both sixteen again! If your sex life has been lagging, working as a "Sex Duet" will certainly give you a jump-start on meeting your physical and emotional goals; your engines will be roaring as they should be! Gradually, you'll be celebrating your fantastic achievements.

You will both be having fun together, and indulging in each other. The best part of all is that both of you will look better and also feel closer.

Here is what one young lady, Amanda, wrote to me after she and her partner followed my personal advice to go on the Ultimate Sex Diet:

Six weeks ago I thought that I was too busy to work out. I had difficulty balancing work, school, and my relationship. On top of all that, I was feeling out of shape and unattractive, and this made me uninterested in sex. But then you told me about the Ultimate Sex Diet, and after just a few weeks of following it, I'm a new woman! My man and I have grown closer than ever. In fact, he's never been happier to support me in a goal. I've improved the muscle tone in my thighs, butt, and stomach, and for the first time in years I have toned arms! We've both made an effort to eat healthier, and he's happier than ever that it's part of my diet to let loose in the bedroom! Now finding time to work out is the least of our worries. The only problem we have is that we'd rather stay in bed on weekends than go out with friends!

Now finding time to work out is the least of our worries. The only problem we have is that we'd rather stay in bed on weekends than go out with friends!

Following the Ultimate Sex Diet as a "Sex Duet" will be even more beneficial because a loving relationship not only leads to better sex; it also enhances the feeling and impact of the growing intimacy between the two of you. According to Dr. Dean Ornish, author of *Love and Survival: The Scientific Basis for the Healing Power of Intimacy*, research has consistently shown that "anything that promotes feelings of love and intimacy is healing." If you have someone who really cares for you and whom you care for in return, someone you are intimately connected with in every way—emotionally, physically, and intellectually—then you will be much less at risk of premature death and disease.

> If you have someone you are intimately connected with in every way, then you will be much less at risk of premature death and disease.

Part of this has to do with the positive effects of touch, which virtually changes the chemical composition of our bodies. Caressing, hugging, stroking, and cuddling send chemical signals to your brain that this is pleasurable, nurturing, and good. In one study conducted in the early 1930s, Dr. Rene Spitz, an attending physician at a number of nurseries for newborn babies, noticed that the illness and mortality rates were substantially higher in certain nurseries. Through his observations and experiments, Spitz found that many of the babies were becoming ill

> When everyone sees the love you have for each other, especially as you slim down and tone up, you'll be the envy of all your friends!

and dying at those nurseries—not because of poor hygiene or nutrition, but rather, because they were not being held and hugged by the nursing staffs. He confirmed his findings by hiring "grandmothers" to come into those nurseries to hold and cuddle the babies. Immediately, the infant illness and mortality rates declined rapidly. So be sure to be affectionate with your partner. Touch them lovingly and often. Not only in private, but also in public! Encourage each other with displays of affection in any place where it is not considered inappropriate. Hold hands, snuggle, and kiss! It is playful and fun for both parties and strengthens the bonds between you. When everyone sees the love you have for each other, especially as you slim down and tone up, you'll be the envy of all your friends!

With your newly awakened, sensual self-image and cuddly closeness, plus the erotic foods you will be eating and the lusty exercises we will discuss, you will soon desire sex more frequently, if not incessantly, which is exactly our goal!

Now, we will move on to discuss specific activities you can both engage in to support and encourage each other throughout the day. Obviously, some of these may not be practical for all of you, depending on your schedules or whether you have children or an elderly parent living with you. However, we encourage you to participate as much as possible.

To begin, keep track of the exercises you perform each night (sexual and otherwise). Remember them the following morning. Recount all the sensual details, including the massages or foreplay prior to intercourse and the various positions you explored. Both of you should also keep track of the foods you ate that day.

Do not be afraid to discuss your sexual fantasies or the activities you can do to heighten each other's arousal and climax.

The following day, when one or both of you are at work, try to set aside ten to fifteen minutes to talk on the phone when you are both able to offer your full attention to each other. At that point, recount the activities you engaged in the night before, and make plans for the upcoming evening. What will you have for dinner, and most importantly, for dessert?! A great suggestion, if you have the opportunity, is to cook your meals together in your underwear, or in even less clothing on occasion. Just be sure to avoid frying foods in the nude. It's dangerous and fried foods are bad for your health!

Do not be afraid to discuss your sexual fantasies or the activities you can do to heighten each other's arousal and climax. Ask your partner if there's anything you can do to provide a more wonderful experience. Perhaps the "oil" (lubricant), the location, or the positions need to be changed. Don't forget, the customer (your partner in love) is always right!

> Discuss "stepping up the pace" to slim down even more quickly.

Another suggestion is to redecorate your bedroom so that it creates a more romantic atmosphere. Simply add a few sexy touches such as sensuous sheets, candles, and soft rugs. Clear out any clutter that may be distracting to the fun at hand.

If someone has to be away on business, or for any reason, set aside a time each night to have a romantic conversation, or even engage in "phone sex" if you're comfortable with it. This extra little boost should excite you, and keep you in the right frame of mind to succeed on the Ultimate Sex Diet.

At the end of each week, weigh yourselves. You can do so privately if you don't feel comfortable having your partner know exactly how much you weigh. Calculate how many pounds you lost by having more sex, exercising moderately, and eating more sensibly. Discuss "stepping up the pace" to slim down even more quickly. Keep a soft shag rug in the bedroom by the scale to "celebrate" your progress or to "make up" for any lost ground in your battle of the bulge.

Additionally, record positive observations about the changes in your partner's body. Make sure to notice and compliment the traits and physical attributes that they find most appealing about themselves and that you feel are most attractive. Give your partner at least three compliments each day.

Since we do not live in a perfect world and we are not

perfect people, it's virtually certain that there will sometimes be disagreements or even fights between you and your partner. This does not mean, however, that your "Sex Duet" is ruined or that both of you will now have to "go solo." This is a time to be especially sensitive to your partner. Use the old trick of counting to ten before you say anything negative. Keep counting until the urge to "put down" is put down. Try to see the situation from your partner's perspective before you react. Avoid insults and harsh words. If a fight does break out, you are required to apologize to each other, and then to participate in make-up sex. Whoever is determined to be at fault must reward the other person with a special session of massage or other pleasure. If the one at fault cannot be determined, the acts of pleasuring must be mutual. Never, ever, get so angry at each other that someone sleeps on the couch or in a different room. Never go to bed angry. It's important to share a bed and to bond, at least through cuddling, each and every night.

> Give your partner at least three compliments each day.

> It's important to share a bed and to bond, at least through cuddling, each and every night.

On every diet, we also encounter difficult days. Some days, dieting is a piece of cake. On other days, you can't help yourself, and you eat the piece of cake. If one partner is having a bad day on the Ultimate Sex Diet, it is up to the other person to encourage them to get back on the program. This is positive reinforcement we are talking about here. Chubby Hubby is an ice cream flavor, not a phrase that should be used to berate your husband. Talk about how great his (or her) body has been looking and how wonderful the experience has been so far. Discuss the bedroom treats that may be in store when your partner gets back on the diet. Finally, verbalize your love for your partner, then give him or her a great big kiss and hug!

Your bond with your partner will be immensely strengthened as a Sex Duet. Sex is not just sex. It is an important part of maintaining intimacy with each other, and one of the most important glues that cement your relationship. Many people fall into the rut of less and less lovemaking; without even realizing it, their life together often quickly follows suit. Keeping your creative energy alive behind closed doors will open new doors in your marriage, or perhaps pry open those that have been locked for years.

> Keeping your creative energy alive behind closed doors will open new doors in your marriage, or perhaps pry open those that have been locked for years.

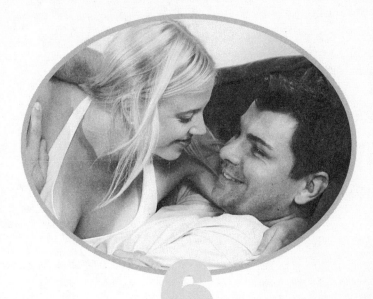

6

LOST AND FOUND:
IGNITING MUTUAL DESIRE

Kissing is nature's way of opening the door to the sexual experience . . . [it is] an exciting excursion into the sensual. If we happen
to be connecting with someone we care about, it produces a sense
of well-being and a kind of full-bodied pleasure . . . It stops the buzz
in your mind, it quells anxiety, and it heightens the experience of
being present in the moment.

—Joy Davidson, Ph.D., psychologist, WebMD.com, January 23, 2004

One of the difficulties of maintaining an active sex life is the need to have a willing partner at the moment when you're in the mood. There is the added complexity of dealing with another person's schedule and mood swings. Sometimes one partner is in the mood when the other is not, then the situation reverses. This can certainly lead to feelings of hurt and pain. Often when this happens, one or both partners feel rejected. Resentment can build, leading to even less sex. Sometimes it reaches the point where the entire topic of making love becomes taboo. That can disastrously lead to a situation where there is little or virtually no sexual activity left in the relationship. Therefore, we should discuss how to seduce a partner, recover long-lost lust, and bring back the desire that used to be there—even if your partner is uninterested at the moment.

This lack of interest in sex is very different from the start of relationships, when there is usually a "honeymoon period." In the beginning, the thrill of the unknown, along with the daydreaming about your new love's body and your partner's desire for you, keep the sex steamy. But most of us have learned, often painfully, that it takes constant effort and commitment to each other to keep the passion going strong. Faced with that challenge, many people just give up on their sex lives. One key to maintaining passion is to continuously reinvent ourselves as we get older—to keep ourselves fresh and interesting to our partners, and most importantly, to ourselves.

Depending on the seriousness of your partner's lack of interest in sex, there may be several strategies that can quickly straighten out the problem. If you partner isn't in the mood for sex, a sensual massage can often do the trick. What about a foot massage, or a bath together lighted only by candles? Men, take your fingers and gently run them through your woman's hair. She'll love the attention and will feel amazingly more attractive. Women, why not give your man an intimate massage or a slow, private striptease? Erotic songs or movies can also work well. Subtle petting, or even passionate kisses at surprising moments, are also effective ways to break through the ice.

An interesting finding came out of a study conducted by Linda Banner, Ph.D., a sex therapist and researcher associated with Stanford Medical School. That study focused on sixty-five couples that had one or both partners who were experiencing sexual dysfunction or lack of arousal. As reported by DiscoveryHealth.com, the study determined that, for 65 percent of the couples, the viewing of educational sex videos was all that was needed to jump-start stagnant sex lives and resume normal marital relations.

If your partner is still not in the mood, you may be able to complete the seduction by kissing him or her everywhere (and

I mean everywhere). Your partner's mood may quickly change. If you are not feeling sexy at the moment, but your partner is, ask for a sensual massage while you lustily describe a secret fantasy. It may actually arouse you and cause you to be in the mood for love as well.

It is important at such difficult or awkward periods to try to recreate the settings in which the two of you were most passionate about each other. Go away for a night or two to a place with special memories or to a hotel or inn to create new ones.

The important thing is to make a considerate, valiant effort to say yes to sex when your partner desires you, even if you may not feel completely aroused at the moment.

The important thing is to make a considerate, valiant effort to say yes to sex when your partner desires you, even if you may not feel completely aroused at the moment. If you accommodate your partner's needs, your partner will be more likely to reward and please you when you are most aroused. What you should not do, however, is go through the motions without putting some creativity, effort, and genuine joy into your lovemaking.

Variety is the spice of sex life! Always keep the salt and pepper (and jam, chocolate syrup, and low-fat whipped cream) handy. Although the missionary position may be the easiest position for you, it may not be the most erotic one. It is fine to use the missionary style time and again, but be sure to also explore new approaches. You can even try the subtle difference of the man rocking back and forth on the woman in this position, rather than simply penetrating in and out. Gently using a little extra pressure with his pelvic bone and rocking back and forth can stimulate the woman's clitoris and heighten

Variety is the spice of sex life!

her arousal. Another variation of this position is to have the woman put her legs together while the man straddles her in a crouching position. All it takes is a slight alteration in technique and the fireworks can begin again.

It is important to continue to grow sexually as a couple. The focus of our lives is largely on our own personal growth: Am I happy? Am I moving forward in my career? Am I making more money? At the beginning, the growth of our relationships with our partners is usually also a major concern. We strive to move forward with one person. We analyze whether we are growing closer and more intimate with our mate. We constantly discuss where the relationship is going, whether we're both happy, and what we can do to improve the relationship and turn it into a lifelong commitment. With time, however, and often simply because a pact has been made to stay together forever, we lose focus on whether the relationship is still developing and what can be done to improve it.

> A committed, long-term relationship is one of the central pillars of our lives . . . We change jobs, houses, and cars, yet in this whirling kaleidoscope we tend to forget the importance of what should never change.

However, our lives don't stop changing once we enter a committed relationship and neither does the life of our partner. Often our lives become significantly more complicated as we deal with life events, and the balance in our priorities shifts. Spouses are taken for granted and feelings are ignored. We stop making the effort to do things as a couple, and we lose our sense of creativity. We stop touching each other the way we used to touch. We don't kiss and hug with our earlier passion. Personally, I think this is very ironic. A committed, long-term relationship is one of the central pillars of our lives. We make very few decisions that entail a lifelong commitment, but once the "honeymoon period" is over, many people forget about the relationship's true significance. We change jobs, houses, and cars, yet in this whirling kaleidoscope we tend to forget the importance of what should never change.

Since we are committed to keeping our partners for the rest of our lives, shouldn't we try as hard as possible to make them happy and keep our relationship with them in the best condition? If you knew that your house or apartment would be the only place you would live in for the rest of your life, would you ignore it and not clean it for weeks? Would you damage the walls or stop improving it? Of course not. You would want to be sure it remained in top condition, so you would maintain it properly for as long as possible, in order to enjoy it for years to come. The same approach should be followed with our partners. Since we hope to have eternity to spend with the love of our lives, we should treat him or her as respectfully as possible and focus on our partners' happiness so that they continue to feel and act like the wonderful people they are. We should continue to cater to them and treat them with the loving care and respect they deserve. Most likely, our partners will reciprocate our love and caring with the warmth and affection that each of us desires.

Now, if the desire to engage in intercourse is missing, what do we as the lustful partner do to change that? Believe it or not, the first step to re-igniting your sex life does not begin with candles, lubricants, or lingerie. It begins with communication. The lack of libido could be due to a number of factors; as partners in life, you can often identify the root causes of the lack of desire by communicating openly and honestly with each other.

Perhaps the lack of desire stems from the resentments built

up over years of minor squabbles, or maybe it stems from the hurt your partner feels because of what you have or haven't done to help him or her. Perhaps your partner just lacks the creativity to conjure up sexual fantasies in his or her mind and needs your help. Talk. Have a heart-to-heart conversation. Be sure not to complain or blame your partner if there is a lack of sex. Instead, turn it around and ask what you can do to make your mate happier. Talk about your relationship and what needs to be done to bring it to the point where you will both be happy. An outstanding sex life will return naturally when you make your relationship a loving and understanding one, and when each of you is the other's top priority.

> An outstanding sex life will return naturally when you make your relationship a loving and understanding one, and when each of you is the other's top priority.

Partners play an important role in arousal; both of you are responsible for creating an atmosphere of love, support, mutual trust, and intimacy. One recommendation is to start focusing on touching rather than sex. If there is a serious lack of desire within your relationship, consider a mutual agreement that you will not have sex with your partner for a few days, a week, or even two weeks. Return to the early days of your life together, before sex was part of your relationship. Spend the time to retrace and re-enact the steps that led to your passionate desire to make love. The "everything but sex" approach can awaken new sensitivities and passions that have dried up long ago.

Go on dates. Take walks in the park. Spend an evening just kissing, without any pressure to have sex or to "take it to the next level." Leave your clothes on and just caress and hold each other. Be playful and touch your partner's cheeks, rub your noses together, and make all the playful little gestures that were so much fun when you first fell in love. Take a moment to really look at each other again. Remember what it was like when you first kissed and how exciting it was before sex was even a part of your relationship.

The next night, continue again, but allow some touching above the clothes. Each night make a little more progress, until you have reached the point of heavy petting that leads to heavy breathing and passionate desire. If you do this correctly and just advance one small step further each night, or move up "one base" as we used to say in high school, you'll be craving the full experience by the time you get there and you will both enjoy it more than you have in years.

Of course, sometimes outside factors are behind the loss of sexual desire. Prescription medications for conditions that are unrelated to sexual activity may be part of the problem. For both men and women, there are a wide variety of prescription medications that can affect our ability to function sexually, such as blood pressure drugs, antihistamines, antidepressants, and ulcer drugs. Consult your physician to determine if one of the medications you are taking could be having a negative impact on your libido. If one of the drugs may be depressing your interest in sex, ask your doctor if there is another version of the drug that does not have the same side effects.

Sexual dysfunction also arises from a number of other causes. For men, erectile dysfunction (ED), or what is often labeled as "impotence," is the repeated inability to achieve or maintain an erection during intercourse. It may be a complete inability to attain erections, an inconsistent ability to achieve them, or the ability to attain only brief erections. According to the National Ambulatory Medical Care Survey, for every 1,000 men in the United States, 7.7 physician office visits were made for ED in 1985. By 1999, that rate had nearly tripled to 22.3. Since that time, erectile dysfunction has become widely discussed and addressed, especially since the introduction of Viagra and other related drugs that target ED. Urologychannel. com reported that the incidence of ED increases with age. Chronic ED affects about 5 percent of men in their 40s and 15–20 percent of men by the age of 65. Temporary ED and inadequate erections affect as many as 50 percent of men between the ages of forty and seventy. It is important to note that ED can be treated at any age. You are never too old to try to seek help for your ED situation!

According to experts, medical conditions cause 90 percent of erectile dysfunction that is not the result of medications or surgery. Such medical causes include blood vessel disorders involving the pelvis and penis, forms of diabetes that affect the pelvic nerves, hormonal disturbances, kidney disease, multiple sclerosis, and many others. Surgery, particularly of the prostate gland or the bladder, can injure nerves or arteries near the penis and also cause ED.

Being overweight can also result in sexual dysfunction. When researchers at the Duke University Diet and Fitness Center studied the sexual impact of weight loss on seventy participants, they discovered that moderate weight loss of ten to thirty pounds significantly improved the libidos, sexual functioning, and satisfaction of both men and women. In a study of one hundred obese men with ED, published in the Journal of the American Medical Association in June, 2003, it was discovered that nearly one-third of the men regained normal sexual function after participating in an intensive weight loss program.

Psychological or emotional factors cause the other 10 percent of ED problems. Feelings of anxiety, guilt, depression, low self-esteem, and fear of sexual failure can all lead to ED. Men who have ED as a result of a medical condition often experience these negative feelings as well. Experts often treat psychologically-based ED by focusing on possible anxiety problems. The patient's partner can help with the remedial exercises, which include the development or renewal of intimacy and stimulation. If ED is a problem, I recommend a medical consultation with an expert in this field. There is nothing to be embarrassed about, and it is important for both you and your partner to make sure the condition is properly treated.

Now, turning to the other member of your Olympic team, medical sexual disorders among women are more complicated and less understood. With men, the focus is primarily on the ability to become erect. Once men become erect, they can usually achieve orgasm. With women, on the other hand, there are three stages that must take place in order for orgasm to occur. According to Robert Griffith, M.D., there must be desire (libido), excitement (arousal), and wetness (lubrication) of the genitals before the games can begin.

Experts estimate that up to 50 percent of all American women experience sexual dysfunction and that up to two-thirds of these women are unable to achieve "the big O." Most of the time, the causes are psychological rather than physical. Although these problems can happen throughout a woman's sex life, apparently they are less frequent as women get older, which is the opposite with men. The current professional consensus is that women age better sexually than men. That's a tremendous relief for me!

Earlier, we discussed how to increase sexual desire. Once the desire is in place, arousal can happen. This involves increased blood flow to the pelvic area, while the vagina actually expands, and the clitoris has a small erection. The increased blood flow causes the secretion of clear mucous fluid, the natural female lubricant, making intercourse smoother and more pleasurable. It is important that this lubrication process be complete before the man enters the woman or the woman's experience can be incredibly painful and cause soreness. So taking the time to have provocative foreplay is essential. As women get older, lubrication may diminish because their vaginal walls get thinner. A variety of health disorders and medical treatments, including diabetes, high blood pressure, and radiation treatment for cancer, can make the problem worse. With a doctor's advice, lubricants such as Astroglide, K-Y Jelly, and even saliva can be used to smooth things along.

So if you do not let the equipment get rusty, it will function like a well-lubricated "love machine" well into your senior years.

Many doctors now believe that the medical complications associated with low sex drive in women are sometimes caused by hormonal deficiencies. The good news is that such deficiencies can be treated with medications. Depending on the problem, some women may need to take testosterone, estrogen, or the female equivalent of Viagra. You need to consult your physician to learn what is best for you. Remember, ladies—the more sex you have, the less likely you are to have these sexual difficulties, so if you do not let the equipment get rusty, it will function like a well-lubricated "love machine" well into your senior years.

Imagine how much fun it will be to reignite your mutual desire. Half the fun is working on the cure!

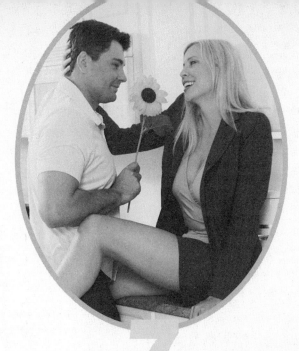

SEXERCISE: TRAINING FOR THE BEDROOM OLYMPICS

Exercise is good and sex is exercise.

—Dr. Fluer Sack, M.D.

You're burning calories and it beats the heck out of jogging.

—Eva Ritvo, M.D., Head, Department of Psychiatry

Mount Sinai Medical Center, Miami Beach

Miami Herald, February 13, 2003

In prior chapters, we discussed a number of ways to increase sexual desire. However, we saved one of the best ways to boost libido for last. No, not Love Potion #9, as the famous "oldies" song suggests. It's exercise.

Exercise helps keep your heart healthy, your body slim, and your brain humming. Studies have shown that exercise also acts as a powerful aphrodisiac. According to Catherine Hood, M.D., an honorary clinical lecturer at Oxford University in England, quoted on Discovery-Channel.com, "[M]oderate regular exercise will help to improve blood flow to the sexual organs. In addition, exercise helps you feel good about yourself. Anything that improves self-esteem will improve libido." DiscoveryChannel.com also reported that the endorphins released by the brain during exercise produce feelings of exhilaration and may release hormones that power the sex drive. It cited research that shows that "women who exercise regularly tend to have more active sex lives, are more easily aroused, and reach orgasms more quickly than those who don't work out."

Exercise helps keep your heart healthy, your body slim, and your brain humming. Studies have shown that exercise also acts as a powerful aphrodisiac.

Of course, different types of exercise programs help build endurance, strength, or flexibility. If you follow the recommendations made in this chapter, and in Chapters 8 and 9, you will improve all three. In this chapter we will emphasize aerobic and cardiovascular conditioning, which will improve your endurance and also boost your libido. Chapter 8 will teach you the exercises you can do before making love to get you toned up and in the mood. Chapter 9 highlights the exercises that can be done during sex to increase your strength and flexibility.

While sex is a fantastic, convenient, and pleasurable way to exercise, moderate exercise outside of the bedroom is also incredibly important. Physical activity increases the speed at which you can reduce your weight because it burns additional calories. Exercise is also needed in order to tone the body's muscles. If you do not exercise while you are on a diet, you may not get the fit, attractive appearance we all want. Therefore, exercise should be a key part of your diet program if you're aiming to look truly fabulous.

Interestingly, moderate exercises that take longer are better than short, intense activities when you are trying to lose weight because you are more likely to burn fat during longer exercise sessions. More intense activities also carry a greater risk of injuries and other stresses on your body. For example, the cardiovascular benefits of fast walking are about the same as those obtained from jogging, but jogging is more likely to result in injury. Also, if you get injured, you will not be able to exercise as much as before or possibly at all; therefore

> **While sex is a fantastic, convenient, and pleasurable way to exercise, moderate exercise outside of the bedroom is also incredibly important.**

choosing brisk walking over running is one way of making sure you can stay on your exercise program for as many years as possible.

As a point of reference, here are some examples of the calories burned doing an hour of various exercises. For a 150-pound person exercising for an hour, walking at a pace of three miles per hour burns 120 calories per half hour; jogging at a pace of seven miles per hour burns 460 calories per half hour; swimming at a pace of twenty-five yards per minute burns 140 calories per half hour; singles tennis burns 200 calories per half hour; and fast-paced dancing burns 200 calories per half hour.

> On this diet, the combination of more sex, additional moderate exercise, and sensible eating may give you and your partner another decade of happy, healthy living to enjoy with each other.

In addition to weight loss, there are countless other health benefits to exercising. Edward Laskowski, M.D., a codirector of the Sports Medicine Center at the Mayo Clinic in Rochester, Minnesota, outlined several of them. First, exercise is good for the heart. It strengthens the heart and may help you live a longer and healthier life. Moderate exercise is also beneficial for your blood pressure. In fact, several studies have reported that it may be better at reducing high blood pressure than more intense exercise. Physical activity is also good for your mental health because it releases endorphins, which boost your mood and reduce stress, depression, and anxiety. Many studies have shown that exercise may also increase your life span. On this diet, the combination of more sex, additional moderate exercise, and sensible eating may give you and your partner another decade of happy, healthy living to enjoy with each other.

BEFORE YOU BEGIN

➤ Always get your physician's approval before beginning a new exercise or diet program,
since any such program may involve risk.

➤ If you're just beginning a fitness program, remember to
comfortably and gradually work up to the suggested frequency
and duration of the exercises.

➤ Practice the partner sexercises wtih someone you know and trust,
and with whom you feel free to communicate. Perform the moves
slowly and carefully, according to your own capacity, and be especially cautious if one partner significantly outweighs the other.

➤ If you ever feel pain, breathlessness, or discomfort,
please stop the exercise immediately.

Exercises You Can Do Together

TAKE A WALK TOGETHER. A lovely walk in a park or down a tree-
lined sidewalk during sunset can be a stimulating aphrodisiac.
It is also the perfect opportunity to communicate; you can con-
verse while walking and catch up on the events of the day.
Strengthening the bonds of your relationship is the ultimate
aphrodisiac.

DOUBLES TENNIS. Playing tennis together can certainly lead to a
grand slam! The sport can be quite fun, even if you're not yet
ready to win the U.S. Open. If you're playing doubles, it's also a
great time to build your teamwork skills, and the men have to
love those short tennis skirts!

YOGA. Yoga is an excellent way to increase your flexibility. This is the perfect supplement to the Ultimate Sex Diet because some of the positions we recommend definitely require body bending. Yoga can also help relax your mind and relieve the stresses of your day so you can better enjoy your private time together.

COUPLES' GYM TIME. Take a trip to the gym together, preferably to your home gym, and exercise on treadmills or stationary cycles. To stay on the same wavelength, you can even bring portable CD or MP3 players and listen to the same sexy music together as you work out. *Don't you love how your partner's muscles move under the spandex?*

TAKE A BIKE RIDE TOGETHER. This can be a very romantic, fun-filled activity and also a wonderful exercise. Just bike around the block like when you were kids, or enjoy a longer ride around the neighborhood. Take a picnic lunch and ride to a beautiful park, river, or beach. Go on a longer ride and stay at an intimate inn for the night.

HORSEBACK RIDING. Once you get the required instruction, you'll find horseback riding is especially effective for working out the inner thighs. It is also quite a bonding experience. *Continue exercising your inner thighs when you get home that night. Giddy up!*

CANOEING OR KAYAKING. These activities are great for working the arms as you tour around a body of water before you tour around your lover's body. Make sure to bring your life jackets. But don't get too frisky in a canoe! Leave the lovemaking for dry land!

PADDLEBOATING. This is another romantic activity that is an outstanding workout for your legs and that you can enjoy together.

SKIING. I'm not a skier because I hate being cold. For those of you who enjoy being outdoors during the winter season, skiing is an adventurous way to exercise and is particularly good for your legs. Try to wear slim-fitting ski clothes so you look more like a snow bunny or an Olympic speed skier than the abominable snowman.

AEROBICS. Many excellent aerobic videos are available. Doing a half hour of aerobic exercise together while watching a workout video can be great fun for you and your partner. Plus, if you're both in very sexy exercise outfits or in your underwear, watching each other exercise can be quite a turn on!

DANCING. Dancing is great for burning calories. It's fun and can also be used to seduce your mate. Most forms of active dancing will burn calories. When you are moving to the beat of your favorite music, you won't even realize that you are giving your body a workout. Prior to making love, spend twenty minutes dancing like crazy dance machines. Dance to a wild tune that you both enjoy—one that makes each of you feel sexy. Move your legs as much as you can. I also suggest learning a few belly-dancing moves. Not only do they look quite seductive; they also work out your stomach muscles and tone your hips and pelvis. Rent the film *Dirty Dancing* and dance close. Really close. If you get too hot while you're dancing, please feel free to remove some of your "stifling" clothes.

> If you get too hot while you're dancing, please feel free to remove some of your "stifling" clothes.

8

SEXERCISE:
FOREPLAY AND FLOOR PLAY

Use the greatest piece of fitness equipment ever created: a bed.

—Zachary Veilleux, *Men's Health*, October 2000

Exercise, exercise. We all realize we need to exercise to get healthy and stay healthy. We understand it will help us get toned, lose weight, and stay slimmer. We also know exercising can be time-consuming (heading down to the gym used to cost me half a day), painful, and boring, boring, boring.

I have a better idea. Besides just huffing and puffing (and getting really sweaty) on some cold, metallic machine or constantly hitting the street on a run or a walk to nowhere, make love. Make lots of love. It'll be much more fun huffing and puffing on the warm, inviting body of the one you love than pumping metal or pounding pavement. You may still get all hot and bothered, but it will be worth each and every sweaty minute. This is one "gym" without monthly fees, long lines, and certainly without a dress code.

Exercising through sex is rewarding on many levels. Some of the rewards are wonderfully obvious. Others require a little focus and effort. If you use the right positions while making love, you can tone, shape, and strengthen nearly every part of your

This is one "gym" without monthly fees, long lines, and certainly without a dress code.

body. The sexy exercises on the Ultimate Sex Diet will focus on improving your arms, legs, stomach, back, and buttocks. We will suggest several exciting new sexual positions that will specifically target these areas. You will find that the best part of toning your muscles while making love is that when you tense specific muscles, the physical sensations are actually enhanced. The sex and the orgasms become even more intense.

Many people have a hard time believing that you can really increase your muscle tone during sex. Obviously, they have never tried "sexercising." When you put your whole heart into it, you can feel the burning in your muscles before you even reach climax. The dual sensations are amazing. Be sure to keep in mind that the longer the sex session and the more passionate the lovemaking, the more calories you will burn! Therefore, men may want to use the old "gentle pinching" technique to delay climax and keep the blood pumping while they're making passionate love!

The beauty of my tone and tease warm-up sexercises is that they'll improve your physique, quicken your pulse (in more ways than one), and empower you to reach new levels of self-confidence.

This chapter will highlight the exercises you and your partner can do before sex to get you in the mood and also to get you toned up. These simple exercises are incredibly stimulating and will be so extraordinarily exciting for both of you that you may tackle each other on the sidelines before you reach the end zone.

All great lovers know that in order to prolong the pleasure of sex and "keep them coming back for more," one must be in tip-top shape. So before attempting the earth-shaking lovemaking positions in Chapter 9, it is important that you indulge in some toning and teasing foreplay. This will allow you and your lover to get loose, limber, and lustful. By doing the tease and tone warm-up exercises in this chapter, you will develop the necessary strength, stamina, and flexibility to hold your own or anyone else when your sexual desires explode into action.

The beauty of my tone and tease warm-up sexercises is that they'll improve your physique, quicken your pulse (in more ways than one), and empower you to reach new levels of self-confidence. These sexercises have worked wonders for me and my friends. When you do them, you will hardly notice that you're burning calories while strengthening and toning your entire body from head to toe. Most importantly, you and your partner will have loads of (very stimulating!) fun while exercising your pelvis, back, butt, legs, and arms. When you sexercise, your heart rate and blood pressure will get elevated and the blood vessels in your genitals will become primed for action. As a result, your cardiovascular system will benefit and your post-workout sex is sure to be explosive.

Before Making Love: Warm-Ups, Tone and Tease Sexercises

Your ideal exercise routine should include at least twenty minutes of stamina-boosting cardio exercises (see Chapter 7) three or four days a week. In addition to the cardio exercises, you should select several of the warm-up, tone, and tease sexercises described in this chapter and do them for twenty to thirty minutes three or four days a week. They will help you to look and feel great. Choose the exercises you want to do according to your physical condition, personal needs, sexual goals, and available time. I can assure you, they will be well worth it. You and your lover will keep coming . . . back for more. These exercises will get you in your best shape and in the mood for the main courses of lovemaking served up in Chapter 9.

Sexercise Warm-Ups

Exercise 1. You Really Got a Hold on Me!

How would you like to enjoy the most powerful pelvic-shaking, body-quaking orgasms of your life? You can! It's really possible! My husband and I have reached new levels of ecstasy since we've been practicing this basic but important love muscle exercise, also known as Kegels. What is so amazing about this sexercise is that it's ridiculously simple, yet incredibly effective, and can be done almost anywhere, anytime. Although it is performed alone, my husband and I really love watching each other practice.

This sexercise will allow you to condition your primary love muscle, known as the pubococcygeus (PC) muscle. Both men and women have it. For women, the PC muscle runs along the sides of the entrance to the vagina. For men, the PC muscle runs through the perineum and connects to both the anus and the scrotum. Having control over your PC muscle is an incredibly empowering feeling. By strengthening and toning my love muscle, I have gained more control over what I am feeling and I have been able to receive incredible pleasure during intercourse. Regardless of the size of your partner's "machinery," this exercise will make every intimate encounter feel just purrrfect. And for you women worried about being "too loose" after childbirth,

> If you want greater control over your sexual performance, you need to practice this love muscle sexercise.

this sexercise will help you get a solid grip on your love life again.

This sexercise is also very important for men because it can help them control the timing of their ejaculation. Practicing this love muscle sexercise can often help men last long enough to satisfy the most demanding lover. The longer you delay ejaculation, the more intense your orgasm will often be when you ultimately blast off. My husband swears by these Kegels, and I second that motion!

As devoted practitioners of this sexercise, my husband and I weren't surprised when we read the results of a study summarized in the Summer 2000 issue of *Urban Male* magazine. In that study, 178 Belgian men with minor erection problems were given a four-month program in which these Kegel exercises were part of their daily routine. When the study was completed, 74 percent of the men involved showed improvement in their erections and 43 percent were completely cured. I am sure their wives and girlfriends are much happier now.

Whether you're male or female, if you want greater control over your sexual performance, you need to practice this Love Muscle sexercise. It only requires a minute of your time. That is an incredibly small price to pay for a huge sexual return.

How to Do It

You do not have to be on the staff of Harvard Medical School to find your PC muscle. It can be found rather easily by simply contracting the muscles that hold back your urine, and then releasing them as if you are trying to force your urine out. Inhale as you contract these muscles, then exhale and release the same muscles. Do this sexercise ten to twenty times per session and repeat it.

Exercise 2. Push Up Your Love Life

This is a sexercise that will get your pelvis warmed up and your lower back in shape for the main event. Dressed or undressed, it is incredibly easy and can be done alone or together with your partner. It is a stretching warm-up that will release tension and stress while toning your back, pelvis, abdomen, and buttocks. All you have to do is tighten and then release the muscles in those areas.

How to Do It

Lie on your back with knees bent and feet flat on the floor, hip-width apart, and with your arms at your sides and palms facing down. Inhale and gently arch up your lower back and pelvis.

Exhale, tighten your buttock muscles, draw your abdomen in, and then press the small of your back and pelvis gently down toward the floor.

Repeat five times, rhythmically tightening and releasing the muscles to create a wave-like motion.

Exercise 3. Hang Loose

This is a fun, hand-holding warm-up that you can do with your partner. I prefer doing it in sexy workout wear. If you're more daring, try it in your underwear or in the nude. "Hanging loose" will help release and stretch tight hips and hamstrings (the muscles at the back of your thighs) and help prevent lower back strain. This exercise will get you loose, limber, and toned and allow you to feel as flexible (almost) as an Olympic gymnast.

How to Do It

Stand facing your partner with your legs hip-width apart. Comfortably hold each other's hands. Allow enough distance between the two of you so that you can both bend and hang forward without knocking noggins.

Inhale, then exhale, both slowly folding forward from the hips and placing your hands together on the floor, with one partner's hands resting on top of the other partner's hands. If the back of your legs are tight, bend your knees. Draw your abdomen in (you don't want too much gut getting in the way).

Hang forward comfortably for five breaths, relaxing your neck and shoulders, and allow your head to hang loosely. Come up slowly to a standing position, pulling in your abdomen.

Exercise 4. The See-Saw

Remember how much fun playing on a see-saw was when you were a kid? This is the adult version. When doing this warm-up with your lover dressed or undressed, it gives you a prime opportunity to really touch and see. This sexercise promotes circulation through the pelvis and the internal sexual organs, and increases the flexibility of the pelvis, hips, legs, and shoulders.

How to Do It

Sit on the floor facing each other, with legs comfortably stretched apart and your feet touching, while accommodating each other's levels of flexibility. Try to keep your legs and spines straight. If the backs of your legs are tight, bend your knees as needed. Comfortably hold hands. While holding hands, one partner leans forward and the other leans backward. You are now balancing each other when moving forward and backward just like when you were on a see-saw.

Return to the starting position before reversing direction. Repeat two to four times at a comfortable pace.

Exercise 5. Sexercise Massage

This is a hands-on sexercise to do with your lover that will warm and loosen up your spine. It will get you so relaxed, you'll feel loose enough to let yourself go. Due to the mutual massaging, this exercise promotes intimacy and closeness as a prelude to your lovemaking.

How to Do It

Gently bend your knees while lowering yourself to the floor. Move your toes underneath, flattening them to the floor, then lower your butt to sit on your heels. Slowly bend forward, lowering your torso and bringing your forehead to the floor while keeping your butt on your heels. Your hands are comfortably resting on the floor beside your hips. Your partner, resting comfortably on his knees behind you, should place his palms and fingers on either side of your spine at the lower back. Pressing very gently, he uses his palms to gradually massage up your back to the neck, and then continues downward to the lower back. Be careful to press and massage gently on both sides of the spine, not on the spine itself. Repeat the massage up and down the sides of the spine, then switch positions with your partner.

Toning Sexercises

Exercise 6. Love Squat

This is a hand-holding, relationship-building, and toning exercise that works the legs and butt while building trust between the two of you. It can be done dressed or undressed. It is a fantastic way to improve your leg muscles and increase your lower body strength for those times when you want to get a little more adventurous in your sex play.

How to Do It

Stand facing your partner with your legs shoulder-width apart; comfortably but firmly hold each other's hands. While holding hands, bend your legs and lower your butts until your thighs are nearly parallel to the floor. Remain in this squat position for three seconds. Do not lower your butt below your knees. Do not let go of your partner's hands, otherwise you'll let your lover down—and letting your lover down is never allowed on the Ultimate Sex Diet! While balancing each other, slowly straighten your legs to standing position. Repeat five times, then switch positions.

Exercise 7. Crunchy Kiss

Who would have thought that an exercise we learned in grade-school could give adults of both sexes such a sexy abdominal workout—and the core strength to grab any tiger by the tail (you can take turns being the "tiger"). This is a sexercise that will provide you with the agility and strength to bend and thrust to your heart's content. I have found that if you are going to do this exercise on a hard surface, it is best to be dressed. However, if you have a mat or plush carpeting, doing it in your underwear or in the nude can be fun. I love doing this exercise even more since my husband and I incorporated a terrific, new, added incentive: lots of kisses.

How to Do It

Lie on your back with your knees bent and your hands crossed in front of your chest. Your partner is resting comfortably on his knees at your feet with his hands gently holding down your ankles. Contract your abdominal muscles as you smoothly lift your torso to a sitting position, while your partner continues to gently hold your ankles down. While you're in the sit-up position, lean forward and kiss. Wet kissing and laughing are certainly permitted. Let go of your lover's lips until the next time, and slowly lower yourself back down to the floor. Work up to two sets of ten. Switch positions with your partner.

Exercise 8. Bridging Your Differences

With this exercise you'll have lots of fun, get in shape, and get aroused—all at the same time! It can be done dressed or undressed. You'll enjoy serious eye contact and hand-holding, while developing an appreciation and trust for your lover. This exercise works the abs, the lower back, the hamstrings, and the muscles at the front of the hips (the hip flexors). After all, you want to have flexible hips when it comes time to do your lovemaking dips.

How to Do It

Sit facing each other about three to four feet apart, with your knees bent hip-width in front of you. Place the soles of your feet against those of your partner, while grasping your partner's hands outside of your legs. Then slowly raise and straighten your legs to erect a bridge in the form of an upside-down V. If the back of your legs are tight, bend your knees. Pull in your abdomen. Hold for three seconds. Continue to hold hands while lowering your legs to the starting position. Repeat three times.

Exercise 9. Super-Lover

Amazing lovemaking demands a very strong back, among other physical attributes. This exercise strengthens the back and legs, to help you build the strength and endurance many sexual positions require. It will also improve your posture by strengthening your lower back and reducing the rounding of the upper back. Do this sexercise side by side with your partner, like super-lovers about to take flight.

How to Do It

Lie face down on the floor with your arms extended forward (think Superman taking flight), your palms turned down, and your forehead on the floor. Inhale, raise your arms upward, and simultaneously lift your chest and legs off the floor, keeping your gaze down toward the floor. Ideally, your legs should stay straight and hip-width apart as you lift them up. To protect your lower back, draw your abdomen in, tighten your butt, and keep both hips firmly on the floor. Hold for three seconds. Exhale, lowering your chest, arms, and legs to the floor. Repeat three to five times.

Exercise 10. Chest Press

This is a sexercise that I love doing in sexy workout outfits. Since my husband is bigger and stronger than me, he is always on the bottom and he really enjoys the visuals. A certain degree of trust and strength is required for this Chest Press routine to avoid any problems. This exercise will build up both partners' chests, shoulders, arms, biceps, and forearms. Ideally, it should be done on some type of padded surface or carpet to protect the back and knees.

How to Do It

The stronger, heavier partner should lie on his or her back, with legs straight on the floor. The lighter partner straddles him or her, with knees on the floor, placing hands on either side of the heavier partner's torso, and with arms straight.

The lighter partner lowers and raises his or her body as if doing bent-knee push-ups over the heavier partner. Work up to three sets of five bent-knee push-ups. When you're lowered into the down position, kiss your lover passionately if you feel in the mood.

After the lighter partner completes his or her bent-knee push-ups, he or she remains in the straddle position. The heavier partner then bends his or her elbows 90 degrees and both partners place the palms of their hands, with fingers lined up, firmly against each other's palms.

As the lighter partner leans forward, the heavier partner presses him or her away while straightening his or her arms (as if doing chest presses), then slowly lowers the lighter partner as his or her arms return to the bent position. Work up to five sets of five chest presses.

Teasing Sexercises

Exercise 11. Libido Lifter

This is one of my favorite teasing sexercises, because it always gets a laugh or a rise out of my husband and it really gets me aroused. I strongly recommend doing this exercise in your underwear or in the nude because of the intimacy it creates. Another special aspect of this exercise is that your hands are free to roam as you tone your thighs and hips. Feel free to place your hands wherever you desire.

How to Do It
While you both lie on one side, snuggle up behind your honey's butt, as if you're going into the spoon position. Instead of bending your knees, keep your legs straight. Your hand movements are only limited by your imagination. I know a caress in the right place always motivates me to greater heights. Lift and lower your top leg ten to fifteen times. You can synchronize your leg lifts like Olympic swimmers, or do them one person at a time. Switch positions and repeat with the other leg.

Exercise 12. Elvis Pelvis
This teasing sexercise will help add even more sensual, burning love into your relationship, and also tone your lower back, butt, legs, and arms. When you and your lover do the Elvis Pelvis press naked together, it is guaranteed to get your motors running.

How to Do It
Stand facing your partner, close enough so that your pelvises are touching. Press your pelvis against your partner's for balance, comfortably raising your arms up to the ceiling as though you're saying "hallelujah"; then slowly lean slightly backward, while maintaining pelvic contact. Be very careful not to bend too far backward. Hold for three counts. Return to your upright, starting position. Repeat five times.

Exercise 13. Dirty Dancing

We all know that dancing together and really cutting loose can be great foreplay, especially when you get all hot and sweaty. When I am alone with my husband at home, we love taking off some of our clothes and turning on our favorite dance music. We create a fun, sensual mood with low lights or scented candles. As we dance together, we can feel that each of us is toning the pelvis, butt, lower back, arms, and legs.

Continue thrusting your pelvis and arms back and forward in opposite directions at the same time, while imagining you are having sex. I dare you to keep a straight face!

How to Do It

Stand facing your partner with your knees slightly bent and arms bent in front of you as if you just drew out two six-shooters. Thrust your pelvis back with arms still in front of you, then thrust your pelvis forward as you are swinging your arms back. Continue thrusting your pelvis and arms back and forward in opposite directions at the same time, while imagining you are having sex. I dare you to keep a straight face! Work up to three sets of ten.

Now that you're sufficiently warmed up, you can really cut loose and let it all hang out as you dance and move your bodies to the rhythm of the music.

Exercise 14. Sexy Breath

This is the last sexercise, but it is certainly not the least important. It is the sensual calm before the torrid sexual storm, and I strongly recommend that you do it dressed in as few clothes as possible. It will give you and your lover an opportunity to feel and caress each other and share a unique and intimate closeness. This simple, easy-to-do conscious breathing exercise will raise the primal energy and put you in a physical, sexual position from which it is very easy and natural to go all the way.

How to Do It

The man, depending on his flexibility, can sit with his legs either crossed or comfortably straight out in front of him. The woman sits in his lap with her legs wrapped around his hips. Allowing for your partner's size and comfort level, wrap your arms around each other and place your hands where they feel most comfortable. Maintain eye contact while you inhale and exhale together. Synchronize your breathing so that you breathe in together for five counts, then exhale for five counts. Do three sets of this breathing exercise together. If you want to really power up the sexual energy, you can also do the "You Really Got a Hold on Me" sexercises while in this position.

This simple, easy-to-do, conscious breathing exercise will raise the primal energy and put you in a physical, sexual position from which it is very easy and natural to go all the way.

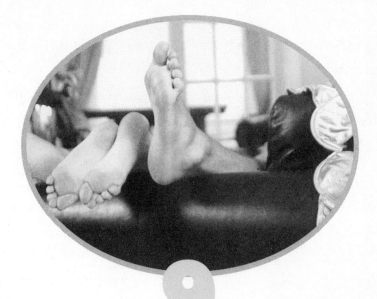

9

SEXERCISE: MORE PASSION
BURNS MORE CALORIES

British model Lisa Snowdon . . . [has] taken a page from [Angelina] Jolie's exercise book. "George [Clooney] and I try to spend as much time with each other as possible. Sex keeps me in shape. I don't diet. I eat what I like. I love Mars bars . . . But what I love best is running off in the middle of the day to make love. It really burns off the calories."

—*Salon*, April 17, 2001

I've heard many people say that if they were given the resources that celebrities have, such as personal trainers and nutritionists, they would be in great shape too. Well, if you follow the Ultimate Sex Diet, consider it done. That's what your partner is: a personal trainer that is with you as you exercise, in and out of the bedroom, and a nutritionist who is constantly monitoring your food intake. Both of you are working as a team. The advantage of using your partner as your trainer and nutritionist is his knowledge of your strengths and weaknesses. Best of all, you do not have to invest in new equipment or new employees. Your partner can use the knowledge of your mutual love to increase the frequency and intensity of your love-making and help you resist the temptations of oversized portions or unhealthy foods. Best of all, both of you have all of the "training equipment" you need to start your personal training program. Presumably you are both well-equipped to participate in sex; if each of you is really well-equipped, all the better!

> Your partner is a personal trainer who is with you as you exercise, in and out of the bedroom, and a nutritionist who is constantly monitoring your food intake. Both of you are working as a team.

Perhaps one of the most important steps to take on the Ultimate Sex Diet is to increase the frequency of intercourse. As mentioned earlier, according to the University of Chicago's National Opinion Research Center, American adults have sex an average sixty-one times per year, or 1.17 times per week. I'm not exactly sure what the .17 entails, perhaps a rather passionate kiss, but at least it takes the average up to more than once a week! Also, as a reminder, sexual activity is 25 percent to 300 percent greater for married couples than for nonmarried partners in most age groups, so all of you "commitment-phobes" out there should take this as a friendly hint to finally settle down! On this diet, we recommend that you engage in intercourse MUCH more frequently than the average couple. In fact, we recommend that you engage in intercourse three to five times during the five-day work week, if you are healthy enough to do so, and twice on either one or both weekend days. This can translate to 1,000–1,800 calories burned per week, depending on the intensity of "the action," if your average lovemaking sessions last for a half hour.

Participating in sex more frequently will increase your life span, in addition to increasing the quality of your life! As discussed above, this was the conclusion of a 1997 article entitled "Sex and Death, Are They Related?" published in the *British Medical Journal*. The report was based on a survey of 1,222 men forty-five to fifty-nine years old from Caerphilly, South Wales. Ten years after the study began, 150 of the men had died. The sexually active group, which included those who had sex more than three times per week, had a mortality rate that was half that of the least sexually active group.

To maximize the health benefits of sex, it is important not

> On this diet, we recommend that you engage in intercourse MUCH more frequently than the average couple.

only to increase the frequency of sex, but also its intensity. So how can you dramatically increase the exercise value of your lovemaking, and what are the best techniques and positions for maximizing the sexual experience? To increase the exercise value of sex, it is important that you both try to tense your stomachs, buttocks, and thighs as often as possible during intercourse. This not only makes these interesting parts of your anatomy seem smaller and more attractive; it also works their muscles and makes them better defined.

> To maximize the health benefits of sex, it is important not only to increase the frequency of sex, but also its intensity.

An effort should also be made to lengthen the duration of your lovemaking sessions. Remember, every additional ten minutes that intercourse is extended burns approximately fifty to eighty more calories. If you find it difficult to extend the amount of time you engage in sex, try switching positions or taking an intermission. Remember, the greatest classic movie epics often had intermissions.

Another technique is to aim for double sessions. Sometimes it is easier to become aroused shortly after one session than to start from the beginning. On weekends, I highly recommend that you take advantage of your free time and double up on at least one of the days.

If either you or your partner has a specific area of the body that needs improvement, try to target that area during sex. Be more creative than just choosing the usual missionary position. Try turning around or squatting, rather than just straddling when you are on top. Also try to stand up, leaning backward or forward to alter the angle of penetration.

> An effort should also be made to lengthen the duration of your lovemaking sessions.

During entry from behind, or what is known as "doggy style," there are many variations that can isolate different muscle groups. For instance, the woman can lean down for more arm pressure to work her triceps, and the man can lift one leg to work his thigh muscles.

You can also increase the intensity of your lovemaking by thrusting (gently!) deeper and deeper. Apply more pressure with your pelvic bones for further stimulation of the woman's clitoris. For those with really creative minds, try different positions that safely involve extra balancing or raising of limbs. Many interesting positions have been documented in recent years in books such as *The Joy of Sex*. For example, the "wheelbarrow" position, where the man is holding the woman's legs while she supports herself on her hands can be a great workout for a coordinated couple in peak physical condition. Another enjoyable position, sure to tone a variety of muscle groups, has the woman lying on her back at the end of the bed with her legs extended straight and her feet resting near her partner's neck. Her partner raises her hips and enters her, working his arms, while she tones her stomach and glutes.

So don't forget to enjoy! Even though sex is being used on the Ultimate Sex Diet as a way to exercise more often, at its core sex is still the ultimate act of intimacy and affection between two people who want to spend their lives loving each other.

There are certainly a wide variety of very satisfying positions to try, and we encourage you to test your flexibility by constantly trying new ones. Use whatever you need: chairs, pillows, rugs, sofas, toys, etc. (I won't ask). Just be very careful not to hurt each other!

Finally, really kiss and hold each other. I was shocked to learn that there are many couples who rarely kiss or show affection during intercourse. They are missing out on so much of what makes lovemaking healthy and intimate. Remember, when you take the sizzle out of a great steak, it's just a piece of meat. So don't forget to enjoy! Even though sex is being used on the Ultimate Sex Diet as a way to exercise more often, at its core sex is still the ultimate act of intimacy and affection between two people who want to spend their lives loving each other.

Some of the Best Sexual Positions for Sexercise

Crouching Tiger, Aroused Dragon

Both partners will quickly realize why the Crouching Tiger has great pleasure and orgasm potential. In this position, the woman does a sexy squat above the man—in a catcher's position. This is the perfect chance for her to use her PC muscles to "catch" his member and clench him tight. The woman can then support herself by putting her hands anywhere on his body for support and then move herself up and down. This also allows the woman to have better control of the depth and pace of the penetration. She can even vary it to tease her partner a little and make sex more interesting. The up-and-down motion may create different sensations than the regular woman-on-top position in which she is lying down in a straddle, moving back and forth. Of course, she will be in better control of her orgasm. If she allows a deep penetration, she can stimulate her G-spot more often. More shallow penetration will touch the edge of the vaginal opening, which is still a pleasurable sensation. Additionally, if the woman leans back, her clitoris can be stimulated. In terms of muscle tone, this position will work her inner thigh and calf muscles. Meanwhile, to get a better view, the man should lift his head and contract his stomach muscles. Maintaining this position as long as possible will give his abdomen a hard work-out. He should feel the tension and clench tighter as it starts to burn. He can even reach forward and caress his partner's body and add to everyone's pleasure.

Down Doggy! Good Doggy!

This erotic, animalistic position is very similar to the usual doggy style, with a few slight changes. After the man enters from behind, as in the regular doggy position, the woman leans down and supports her weight on her elbows, rather than staying on all fours, while the man lifts one bent leg forward, rather than kneeling on both knees. This is highly erotic for the woman because it places direct pressure on her G-spot, which is on the anterior (tummy side) vaginal wall, intensifying her climax. The woman can also maneuver the penetration by slightly arching her back or raising herself a bit. Meanwhile, the man will feel extraordinary sensations in his private parts. This position is also appealing for the change of pace involved in not always looking at each other's face. The woman will feel the tension in her triceps while making love in this position and the man will work his thighs when his leg stays raised. He should switch legs halfway through to hit the G-spot from a different angle.

Stiff As a Board

This is quite similar to the regular missionary position, but it will bring you both to climax sooner. When the man is on her "doing the missionary," the woman extends her legs straight and squeezes them together. This provides more direct clitoral and G-spot stimulation for the woman, and she will also have a

tighter grip on the man, making it more sensual for both parties. The pressure is constant on both the man's and the woman's pelvic regions, and the tightened vaginal area will increase
the arousal of each of the partners. To get into this position, the
man should enter as in the regular missionary style and then the
woman should slide her legs underneath his as he rests his knees
outside her legs. The man will work the muscles in his thighs
and buttocks, while the woman's main focus should be on
squeezing her legs tightly together, tensing her thighs, glutes,
and hips. Done properly, this position should create especially
heightened sensations in her pelvic area.

On a Mission for Pleasure
Of course, the missionary position can also be exciting, fulfilling, and very orgasmic. When the woman wraps her legs around
the man, she should squeeze with her legs as hard as she can,
working her inner thighs. She should also lift her buttocks and
raise herself as the man enters, which deepens the penetration.
A pillow can be placed under her rear to raise her up even
higher and alter the angle of penetration. Rather than lying on
her, the man should stay propped up in a kneeling position to
get better tone in his legs. Additionally, the woman can put her
arms above her head and push on the bed's headboard as the
man thrusts into her.

Humpty Bumpty
In this position, the man is sitting up while the woman is sitting
on him with her legs raised in the air in a straddle. She holds
onto his neck with her hands while he maneuvers her back and
forth. This will work the woman's arms, stomach, and legs.
The man will tone his arms while moving the woman's body,

and will strengthen his legs from the support he is providing to his partner.

Wheelbarrow of Fun

The woman lies on her stomach on the bed with her legs slightly open and her knees slightly off the edge. The man stands behind her at the end of the bed and lifts her legs up toward him, until he is able to enter from behind. The woman then bends her legs and wraps them around him, locking her feet together at the ankles, while the man holds her with his hands and rests her on his thighs. This will tone the woman's triceps, biceps, and stomach, and the man's triceps and lower back. You can also try this on the floor. If you're really talented, you can try walking around the room while in this position and think back to your days in summer camp during color war.

Stand Up and Do It

While standing, the man holds the woman, and the woman carefully uses a bar above her head (such as a very securely fastened chin-up bar), to pull herself up and then down so she can "grab" her partner. She continues doing pull ups while the man is working his arm and thigh muscles by holding her up.

Bend It in the Bedroom

There are a few variations of this position, depending on which leg muscle the woman intends to tone. She can also vary the position during the act and tone all of them. In the first variation, the man sits in a sturdy chair while the woman is standing in front of him, facing him, with her legs on either side of the chair. The woman then does a squat like a ballerina, allowing him to enter. She continues to squat up and down and has complete control of the level of penetration. The man will not get much of a workout in this position, but he can, of course, be flexing his buttocks and contracting his stomach as he lifts himself slightly into her. Another "twist" that can be added to this position is for the woman to twist around and face in the other direction.

Fatal Attracting

This position is reminiscent of the scene in the movie *Fatal Attraction*, when Glenn Close is sitting on the counter while she and Michael Douglas are engaged in wild sex. Doing it spread-eagled on a table while your man faces you to thrust from the front creates mega heat in a minimal amount of time. "He's sure to come quickly because he plunges deep," says Anne Hooper, author of the *Great Sex Guide*. "Plus, men get off on the novelty of doing it somewhere new to them, [since] out of the bedroom equals no-holds-barred sex."

Laid-Back People

Using pillows or bed bolsters, both of you get into a reclined position with the woman on top. The man works his stomach, while the woman works her calves and thighs.

Reverse Cowgirl

This position is the good, old-fashioned, woman-on-top style that begins with the lovers facing each other, but she does the "hokey pokey" and turns herself around so that she faces away from the man. Then he gets on top and does his own "hokey pokey." This works the woman's thighs; she can also tense her stomach. The man should also tense his stomach and lift his shoulders off the bed for further toning.

Let's Get Crazy

This position is a great workout for the woman's stomach and buttocks. While lying on her back, the woman extends her legs straight in the air, slightly spread, with her rear lifted off the ground. The man bends down in a slight squat to enter her, working his quads, and when using his arms for support, he works his triceps.

T-rific!

The woman lies on her side, while the man kneels and straddles her bottom leg perpendicularly (i.e., at a right angle to her, thus forming a terrific "T") and then enters her. Her top leg remains extended upward, gently supported by the man. When done correctly, this can be a great position for deep penetration, while exposing the clitoris for manual stimulation. This double stimulation is very gratifying and can often lead to the big "O" very quickly.

Get a Leg Up

This is a variation of doggy style, where the man enters the woman from behind, but both partners have one leg up off the bed. The leg off the bed can be used to support the movement by pushing off the headboard of the bed. This should work both legs. Switch sides of the bed halfway through to work both legs.

Electric Sliding

Both partners sit on the edge of the bed and the man acts as a slide. The woman essentially sits on his lap while gliding down his body. The man can lean back and support himself with his triceps for extra arm toning and should also thrust up into the woman. This is a leg workout for both the slide and the slider, and much more fun than any plastic playground slide!

"O MY!" THE FEMALE ORGASM

Martine McCutcheon [who starred in the film *Love Actually* opposite Hugh Grant] has revealed that her svelte new look and clean skin is due to "loadsa shagging" with her latest man . . . The 27-year-old . . . has never looked better.

—*London Daily Mirror*, October 15, 2003

Having an orgasm during sex is almost a guarantee for many men. That is probably why they look so content and wistful after making love. Bless their (fully focused) hearts! For women, however, orgasm often does not occur during sex. Even Kim Cattrall, who played the sex goddess character in the television program *Sex and the City*, admitted in her book *Satisfaction: The Art of the Female Orgasm*, that she had an unsatisfactory sex life until she was well into her forties. Many women are unable to achieve vaginal orgasms and are only able to reach climax through stimulation of the clitoris. Depending on the position and technique used during sex, the clitoris is often not sufficiently stimulated for the woman to achieve orgasm.

Having an orgasm during sex is almost a guarantee for many men. For women, however, orgasm often does not occur during sex.

The clitoris is similar physiologically to the penis. When arousal occurs, it fills with blood and has a mini-erection. A woman's orgasm is defined as the point at which all the sexual tension that has been building during her arousal is suddenly released in a series of involuntary and pleasurable sensations and muscular contractions that may be felt in the vagina, uterus, or even the rectum. Of course, not all women who experience orgasms also experience contractions. Some researchers believe that there is just one type of orgasm, clitoral, while others believe there are two different types, clitoral and vaginal, and that each produces different sensations. Those experts who believe in the two types of orgasms claim that during the clitoral orgasm, the vagina lengthens and causes a pocket to form beneath the uterus. During a vaginal orgasm, the uterus drops lower and the vagina shortens. Stimulating both the vagina and the clitoris may cause a possible third kind of orgasm, one that feels different from each of the other two types.

Orgasms are very individual experiences, and there is no correct technique or pattern that must be followed to achieve them. Whatever works for you and makes you feel wonderfully alive, attractive, and happy is the right path to follow.

The first step women must take to achieve orgasm during sex if they are unable to orgasm vaginally is to locate the clitoris. It can be found under the hood at the top of the vagina. Generally speaking, gently caressing or stroking the clitoris during intercourse will increase a woman's potential to achieve arousal and orgasm. However, many of the more traditional sexual positions, such as the missionary position, may not be the best ways for a woman to reach orgasm. This can easily be remedied by manually caressing the woman's clitoris during sex or by using positions that maximize contact with the clitoris and other sensitive areas such as the lips of the vagina and the G-spot.

The clitoris can be stimulated through a number of different

> Many of the more traditional sexual positions, such as the missionary position, may not be the best ways for a woman to reach orgasm.

methods during intercourse. The woman can stimulate herself with her own hand, or the man can use his hand or other (clean!) body parts. Either method can be visually seductive to the other party. Sex toys or vibrators are other alternatives that can add variety and extra stimulation. The man's pubic bone is another excellent tool for arousing the clitoris. If the man focuses on moving back and forth rather than up and down, and presses his pubic bone (not too hard!) against the area of the woman's clitoris, it can be incredibly arousing for her and lead to orgasm. The man should push his pelvis against the woman's groin and maintain a pleasant and consistent pressure, while rocking back and forth or from side to side.

Another recommended method for clitoral stimulation is manual petting or oral sex prior to or following intercourse. If the woman orgasms during foreplay, there is less anxiety and pressure for the man to please her during the act of intercourse, so it can be more enjoyable for both parties. Some women will need a break between orgasms, though others can and want to have several in a row. Sometimes lightning does strike twice (or even more times) at the same spot! For many women, when they have climaxed once, it is much easier to stay aroused and achieve orgasm a second time.

If a woman has never had an orgasm, it does not mean that she should despair of ever experiencing one. There is a specific place inside the vagina named the G-spot (short for the Grafenberg spot, named after the researcher who officially "discovered" it). The G-spot consists of a small bundle of nerves about an inch in diameter and is located about an inch or two inside the vagina on the front wall, or the side closest to the navel. The sensitivity in this region can become extremely heightened when stimulated during intercourse, and the G-spot can even swell.

Sometimes during stimulation of the G-spot, the urethra can even release a clear fluid, similar to that produced by the prostate gland in men. There are reports that about 10 percent of women can actually squirt or ejaculate!

It is important that couples learn the sexual positions that are particularly effective in stimulating the G-spot. In order to help the woman achieve a vaginal orgasm, the man needs to make sure that he is "hitting" the G-spot with each stroke. Several of the sexercise positions we discussed in Chapter 9 are particularly effective for hitting one or more home runs off the Big G Monster.

It can be difficult for a man to know how to stimulate a woman who cannot achieve orgasm on her own. I strongly encourage women to explore their own bodies, so they can show their partners exactly what to do.

Reaching orgasm is wonderful, but if a woman begins focusing on it too much, it can actually become more difficult to achieve. When she gets close to the big "O," if she stops focusing on the enjoyment and sensations she is feeling and only focuses on reaching orgasm, she may not be able to reach it. This can become very frustrating! When this happens, I recommend that she take a step back, stop focusing on having an orgasm, and just concentrate on enjoying the lovemaking. Ironically, when a woman is not trying so hard to orgasm, and is instead soaring in the ecstasy of intercourse, she is more likely to climax.

> I strongly encourage women to explore their own bodies so they can show their partners exactly what to do.

Once the woman has learned to orgasm during sex, it is sometimes possible for both parties to jointly orgasm at the same time. Though having simultaneous orgasms during sex is fabulous, it may not happen very often. Also, do not be overly concerned if the methods suggested above are not working and the woman is not reaching orgasm often enough. Sex can still be very enjoyable. Practice, practice, practice (as if you needed an excuse). The more you practice, the better it will be.

11

USING THE AFTERGLOW

Anything that promotes feelings of love and intimacy is healing.

—Dr. Dean Ornish,
Love and Survival: The Scientific Basis
for the Healing Power of Intimacy

One of the magical rewards of sex is the intimacy and closeness that we feel for our partner after making love. As Victoria Zdrok, Ph.D., a clinical psychologist, jokingly told me, "Sex without love is an empty experience. Of course, it is the most enjoyable empty experience you will ever have." Dr. Zdrok also happens to be the beautiful 2002 Penthouse Pet of the Year. I am sure many men would want to enjoy an empty experience with her (not that she would be willing!). However, the Ultimate Sex Diet is not about empty sexual experiences. It's about having fulfilling, meaningful experiences filled with love and romance. I believe we all want to add more emotional depth to our relationships and sex lives. Therefore,

One of the magical rewards of sex is the intimacy and closeness that we feel for our partner after making love.

we need to focus on how to fully enjoy and benefit from the sweet contentment and intimacy that comes with the afterglow of making love! This is a time when each of us has the opportunity to really embrace our partner and shower them with affection.

Within our body, the release of a hormone known as oxytocin

can be triggered when we have sex. Oxytocin is known as the "cuddle hormone" because it promotes bonding and intimacy. It triggers the physical contractions of childbirth and breast-feeding in women, and orgasms in both men and women. It is also believed to promote social bonding by triggering feelings of warmth and closeness to others. In experiments performed in the 1990s by researcher Dr. C. Sue Carter of the University of Illinois at Chicago, it was shown that when female prairie voles (a type of prairie dog) were injected with oxytocin, they quickly bonded with a single partner. When release of the hormone was blocked, they coupled less avidly and more indiscriminately.

In addition to the oxytocin hormone being released during sex, mood-enhancing serotonin and endorphins are also released. These hormones reduce stress, relax us, and produce the feeling of satiety we experience after making love. While the two of you are in this relaxed state, don't just doze off. Make an effort to have your most intimate conversations. Something to keep in mind, though, is that sex can trigger opposite reactions in men and women. It often has the tendency to put men to sleep, yet stimulate women and wake them up. So here's some advice for the ladies. One way to keep your partner awake and interested is with erotic sex talk. Talk about the seduction leading up to your lovemaking that day or night, and what was fantastic about the position or positions you used. Keep his mind aroused and he will be more likely to give you the postcoital snuggling and say the loving words you are craving. Another technique is to give the man a gentle massage (while avoiding his private areas, which may be overly sensitive

> You can also use the after-sex feeling of intimacy to really open up to your partner and to talk about all of the intimate matters that are on your heart and mind.

at that moment). You can carry the moment into the bathroom and enjoy a shower or bath together. Lovemaking and a refreshing shower together are a great start to the work day, or a beautiful way to end a passionate night.

You can also use the after-sex feeling of intimacy to really open up to your partner and to talk about all of the intimate matters that are on your heart and mind. Ask your mate about what's making him or her happy or how your relationship could improve. Give your spouse the same opportunity to open up and discuss what is on his or her heart and mind. This is also a very good time to talk about sex. Some people are not comfortable broaching the subject at other times, but immediately after making love, they may be more willing. Discuss your fantasies and ask about your partner's desires. What does he or she think about during sex? What can you do to stimulate him or her more? Does your partner want to try love toys, sex foods, or naughty videos? These are the times to really open up.

> To me, there is no better feeling in the world than holding your partner after making love. With your naked bodies touching, it feels like you fit together like the pieces to the mysterious jigsaw puzzle of life.

But please, never, ever criticize your lover after sex and don't discuss topics that will trigger tension or anger. Make sure to give your partner loving compliments about his or her performance and body. The better you make your lover feel, the better he will make you feel. Plus, you'll be more likely to get even more sex!

To me, there is no better feeling in the world than holding your partner after making love. With your naked bodies touching, it feels like you fit together like the pieces to the mysterious jigsaw puzzle of life. After Ben and I make love, the tingling sensation throughout my body and the bond I feel with him are reminiscent of when we first met. Every kiss and touch simply makes me melt, and I can feel my stomach slowly doing flip-flops. I also find that on days when we have sex in the morning, we carry the afterglow and we're more considerate toward each other throughout the day. We also flirt more and are more play-ful with each other than usual. Interestingly, if we have sex in the morning, it is more likely that we will have sex that evening. Perhaps that is because the sweet memories stay on our minds and gently arouse us throughout the entire day.

12

SEXUAL NUTRITION: HEALTHY FOODS FOR HEALTHY LOVING

Eat the right foods. If your body becomes frail due to bad health, sex invariably suffers.

—Catherine Hood, M.D., DiscoveryChannel.com

We all know the phrase "You are what you eat." To me, this phrase never really made much sense because I don't think there is any piece of food I would want to be. Even if I had the choice, I fear that I would rather be a decadent piece of chocolate cake than a boring piece of broccoli. Though you may not actually become the food you eat, you are affected by the nutrients and vitamins (or lack thereof) in what you eat throughout the day. The food has an impact on your mood, your motivation levels, and your body image. *Prevention* magazine reported in August 1991 that researchers have found that fatty foods actually limit the production of testosterone, potentially reducing the sex drive. In one study, men's testosterone levels dropped by 30 percent four hours after they ate a fatty meal. The testosterone levels of men who had healthier meals were unaffected. The same results were also believed to apply to women. Be sure your meals are making you sexier, not less sexy!

Be sure your meals are making you sexier, not less sexy!

On The Ultimate Sex Diet, the foods we recommend are all aimed at keeping you as healthy as possible, making you feel good about your body, and craving nothing but a great bedroom session at the end (. . . and beginning . . . and middle) of the day. This diet is more realistic than many others because you aren't restricted to eating certain types of foods. In fact, you can incorporate into your diet most of the foods you enjoy as long as they are healthy for your body, the portions are reasonable, and you are continuing to gradually achieve your ideal weight and body shape.

> You can incorporate most of the foods you enjoy into your diet, as long as they are healthy for your body, the portions are reasonable, and you are continuing to gradually achieve your ideal weight and body shape.

A common mistake many people make is gorging on their food too quickly. If you're like me, I find there is no bigger turnoff than a gross chewer or eater, so keep this under control. Plus, you may consume more calories if you eat too quickly because it takes between twelve and sixteen minutes for the stomach to transfer signals that it is full to the brain. You certainly don't want to be eating after you are really full.

Eating should be a complete sensory experience, and every aspect of it should be appreciated to its fullest. Before you consume any food or drink, you should set up an environment in which you will be sensitive and aware of every aspect of the experience of eating. Limit your portions. Turn off the television. Treat the food as if you are making love for the first time. Pretend that you are eating it in front of your lover, and that you want to seduce him or her with how sensually you eat your food.

The key is to do everything slowly. The first step is to sit down so you do not feel rushed. Before putting any food in your mouth, inhale its aroma to get your digestive juices flowing. Close your eyes so you can register the scent. Your sense of smell will be heightened on this diet anyway because a better sense of smell is yet another benefit of sex. According to an October 2003 article in Forbes.com, after making love we experience a surge in the production of a hormone called prolactin, which causes the stem cells in the area of the brain that controls the sense of smell to work more effectively.

> Eating should be a complete sensory experience, and every aspect of it should be appreciated to its fullest.

After you have inhaled the aroma of your food, cut it into small, bite-sized pieces. This will make you more aware of how much you are eating and will also ensure that you enjoy each bite of food. You'll naturally wind up eating less. Finally, place the food in your mouth. Keep it in your mouth for a few seconds before chewing to appreciate the taste.

Take your time chewing the food, and feel it with your tongue. Most people do not chew their food well enough, which leads to slower digestion. Masticating is not a dirty word! Consciously chew each bite several more times than you normally would. Chewing breaks up the fiber that holds the food together so that the digestive enzymes have easier access to the nutrients inside. Even the fats in the food get a head start on being digested while they are in the mouth, by receiving a tiny squirt of a fat-digesting enzyme called lingual lipase. When you chew more slowly, you also swallow less air, so you will be less likely to annoy your partner later with smelly burps.

Finally, after you swallow each bite, lick your lips and wait five seconds. Let the after-taste linger before you put another bite in your mouth. Prolong the eating experience as much

> Gradually, you will feel satisfied with smaller portions. This should really help you shed the pounds.

as you can. You may be surprised to find that you become full sooner; you may not even be able to finish everything on your plate. Although you may not be able to eat as much as you previously did, you will feel more satisfied and than ever before. Gradually, you will feel satisfied with smaller portions. This should really help you shed the pounds.

The same approach applies to drinking beverages. Always inhale the scent of your beverage first; register the aroma; and take small, slow sips. Do not slurp, whatever you do! With carbonated drinks (the sugar-free variety, please), you may want to sip slowly; if so, use a straw and it will prolong your enjoyment of the drink. Plus, it can look very sexy if you let the straw dangle between your lips. There should also be no reason for you to ever chew ice. We all know that means you're sexually frustrated! None of that on this diet!

A very sensual technique when you are eating with your partner is to feed each other. The meal will take longer, but you may also get so worked up you don't even finish (the meal that is)!

A very sensual technique when you are eating with your partner is to feed each other. The meal will take longer, but you may also get so worked up you don't even finish (the meal that is)! Chopsticks can also be helpful on this diet. They look quite seductive, and because it will take longer to maneuver your food when using them, you will feel full sooner with less food. After you eat, make sure to do plenty of kissing. Research shows that kissing helps saliva wash away food from the teeth, lowers the level of the acid that causes tooth decay, and prevents the buildup of harmful plaque on teeth.

Many of these techniques can be transferred to the bedroom when you engage in sex. All your senses should be heightened, and every step of the experience should be isolated and appreciated. A good session of lovemaking requires attention to every detail, feeling, and emotion. Every time you have sex, remember that it is a fresh new start to your love life, even though it is happening with the same person. If you love chocolate,

> **Take care not to eat too much right before exercising or engaging in sex.**

you still savor it immensely even if you've eaten it the day before, or even two hours before. You enjoy its sensations every time. That is how sex with your partner should be. Never minimize the experience for yourself or your partner.

Take care not to eat too much right before exercising or engaging in sex. As you may have noticed, eating a large meal before you exercise makes you feel sluggish, tired, or even nauseous. According to Stephen DeBoer, a registered dietician at the Mayo Clinic in Rochester, Minnesota, your body can digest food while you're exercising, but not as efficiently as it can while you are sedentary: "Your blood goes to whatever part of your body needs it. When you start exercising, some blood gets taken away from your stomach. Both jobs get done, but not as effectively or as side effect-free as you'd like." So, take care to leave enough time between when you eat and when you plan to exercise. As you know, on the Ultimate Sex Diet, exercise also includes your activities between the sheets! If possible, try to wait two hours before engaging in strenuous activity after large meals, and about an hour after smaller meals. Little snacks are fine even twenty minutes before exercising.

> **Additionally, make sure to stay well-hydrated throughout the day, particularly on days when you exercise, do heavy work, or sweat profusely.**

On the other hand, working out when you're feeling starved is not a good idea either. Low blood sugar levels can make you feel sluggish, weak, or even light-headed. On this diet, you should only feel light-headed when you are "walking on air" from happiness, not from a lack of healthy foods.

Additionally, make sure to stay well-hydrated throughout the day, particularly on days when you exercise, do heavy work, or sweat profusely. Try to drink about six to eight glasses of water a day, and more if you are exercising, because you lose the critical fluids and electrolytes your body needs when you exercise or engage in strenuous work.

My final recommendation in terms of eating techniques is to make sure to eat breakfast! "Breakfast not only starts your day off right; it also lays the foundation for lifelong health benefits," says Jennifer K. Nelson, director of clinical dietetics at the Mayo Clinic. Studies show that people who eat well-balanced breakfasts actually consume fewer calories during the day than those who skip a morning meal. They also have a healthier, more well-balanced diet and tend to go on fewer eating binges throughout the day. Ideally, I also recommend a nice morning romp. Why shouldn't each of you have the chance to start the day off right (on top)?!

> Ideally, I also recommend a nice morning romp. Why shouldn't each of you have the chance to start the day off right (on top)?!

Good Foods for Making Great Love

An aphrodisiac is a food, drink, or scent that is alleged to arouse or increase sexual desire or libido. Hundreds of food products have been given this label, though it is difficult to prove their efficacy. Some of the more unusual aphrodisiacs include a ram's testicle mixed with honey, goat eyes, and deer sperm. Frankly, it's hard for me to see how you can become more interested in sex if you're eating such unpleasant "foods," especially when they make you want to run to the bathroom instead of the bedroom!

In my opinion, aphrodisiacs work in large part by the power of suggestion. Their impact is similar to the placebo effect demonstrated in many medical experiments in which patients believe they have been given a pill that will relieve them of their pain or symptoms. The patients will often begin to feel expected results, even though they have been given a sugar pill. Similarly, if I tell my husband that if he eats a certain type of food, he will think about my breasts . . . what do you think he'll think about? Of course he will think about the lovelies and most likely get really aroused.

I do believe there are certain "mood foods" associated with romance that can promote feelings of desire. These include combinations like champagne and strawberries, or indulgences like caviar or oysters. Smells associated with certain foods may also trigger memories of past romantic escapades and excite us. Other foods can alter the taste of our body fluids and make oral pleasure more inviting. Finally, there are the obvious phallic shapes that can be suggestive while eating and that will visually stimulate a partner if they have an active (or even not so active) imagination. Of course, we are all individuals with unique tastes and experiences, so there may not be universal aphrodisiacs that apply to everyone. However, let's discuss a list of those foods that many people find erotic. Interestingly enough, many of the foods classified as aphrodisiacs are quite healthy and tasteful.

Below is a list of healthy foods that you should consider including in your diet. Many are vegetables that are phallic-shaped and extremely nutritious. On this diet, you should eat at least six to eight servings of fruits and vegetables a day, but feel free to eat as many green vegetables as you want to during the day. Consumption of starchy vegetables or those containing high amounts of fatty substances, such as avocados, should be limited. I encourage you to make vegetables even more flavorful because steamed or raw vegetables may not always be fully satisfying. There are many options for adding flavor to vegetables without drenching them in fatty salad dressings. Consider sprinkling a bit of salt, soy sauce, salsa, or hot sauce on your veggies. You could also try sautéing them in a dab of olive oil or dipping them in a low-fat dressing. However, before making love I do avoid eating brussels sprouts. Though they are good for you, to me they smell too much like flatulence, which can certainly kill a mood.

In general, I am morally opposed to eating bland-tasting food. I believe that eating foods devoid of interesting or tantalizing tastes will not satisfy your hunger. Even if your stomach is no longer empty, your emotional food cravings may not have been filled. Often people eat bland-tasting food, but later give in to their desires for the tasty, but unhealthy, treats they really wanted to eat in the first place.

Recommended Vegetables

ASPARAGUS. Not only is it phallic-shaped; it's also great for you. Beware though, because it makes semen taste worse.

ARTICHOKE. The soft leafy petals are flavorful and healthy, and subtly resemble the lips of a woman's vagina.

ARUGULA. Arugula or "rocket seed" has been documented as an aphrodisiac since the first century A.D. Incredibly healthy for you, arugula greens are frequently used in salads and pasta.

BEAN SPROUTS. Essentially calorie-free, these sprouts also look like sperm!

CARROTS. It is documented that Middle Eastern royalty has long regarded the carrot to be a significant aid in seduction. Carrots are also reported to improve vision, so you can get a better view of your lovely partner. Just do not eat too many or you may turn orange yourself!

CAULIFLOWER AND BROCCOLI. These veggies are high in nutrients and delicious when sprinkled with lemon juice or a very small dab of butter or cheese.

CELERY. Enjoy! It is low in calories and high in fiber. Sprinkle it with a little salt for extra taste, or dip it in a low-fat dressing. Every stalk is packed with androstenone and androstenol, two pheromones that can help men attract women. According to *Men's Health* magazine, chewing a stalk of celery releases androstenone and androstenol odor molecules into your mouth. These pheromones travel up the back of your throat to your nose and begin to boost your arousal. They also cause your body to send off scents and signals that make men more desirable to women.

CUCUMBERS. Interestingly phallic-shaped, they have a firm enticing texture.

GREEN BEANS. Green beans are great for you. That's the reason the Jolly Green Giant is so tall! Cook them in low-fat cream of mushroom soup, or sprinkle them lightly with lemon juice and slivered almonds and you have a great treat.

MUSHROOMS. Shaped like a head of a man's private parts, mushrooms are low in calories and add a little variety to the mix.

SPINACH AND BEANS. Researchers in Australia, Indonesia, and Sweden studied the diets of 400 elderly men and women, and found that those who ate the most leafy green vegetables and beans had the fewest wrinkles. Spinach and beans are full of compounds that help prevent and repair wear and tear on your skin cells as you get older. The only question is why was Popeye's face so distorted? He did have sexy muscles though.

TOMATOES. Many believe that in the Garden of Eden, it was actually a tomato, not an apple, that Eve offered to Adam. This is why tomatoes are reputed to be powerful aphrodisiacs. Sprinkle them with salt, basil, and a dab of olive oil, and they are simply divine.

Enticing Fruit

Fruits are nature's candy. They are sweet, seductive, and delicious. If you are someone who craves sugar (like me), you will find that fruit is the perfect substitute for cakes, cookies, and candies (interesting how these foods all begin with the same letter as calories). When I am craving gummy bears, if I eat a bowl of strawberries with a packet of artificial sweetener sprinkled on them, I find that my craving is often satisfied. Of course, one should use artificial sweeteners very sparingly because of the health concerns that have been raised about them.

Additionally there's something very sensual about taking a bite of a fruit that has a firm exterior, and experiencing the explosion of sweet succulent juice released in your mouth. Virtually every fruit is packed with vitamins and nutrients. And the slow-digesting carbs in these juicy treats, as well as in whole grains, nonstarchy vegetables such as beans and soy, and low-fat dairy products such as yogurt, offer a steady supply of fuel for energy throughout the day.

However, I do recommend limiting your intake of fruit juices. Fruit juices are high in sugar and calories. It is actually healthier to eat the whole fruit because its fiber is extremely healthy for the digestive system. Finally, try freezing fruits such as grapes or strawberries and eat them as delicious dessert treats. They will take longer to eat, and their frozen consistency makes eating them feel like eating a popsicle.

APPLES. An apple a day may not keep the doctor away, but it has been said to elevate moods and work as an antidepressant. How do you like them apples?

BANANAS. Bananas have a pleasing, phallic shape; they are also rich in potassium and B vitamins necessary for sex hormone production. Additionally, the high content of chelating minerals and an enzyme called bromelain in bananas is said to aid in boosting male erectile efficiency. So eat bananas, and then drive your lover bananas!

BERRIES. Raspberries, strawberries, cherries, and other berries are sweet and delicious. The perfect foods for seductive hand-feeding, they are also high in vitamin C and make a sweet, light dessert. Dip them in a little light or fat-free whipped cream and lick them slowly for further sensual pleasure.

BLUEBERRIES. "These are of the best foods for older men with erectile problems," according to Mary Ellen Carnire, Ph.D., a professor of food science at the University of Maine. "They're loaded with soluble fiber, which helps push excess cholesterol through your digestive system before it can be broken down, absorbed, and deposited along the walls of your arteries. They're also packed with compounds that help relax your blood vessels, improving circulation, which is important for [proper functioning of] the penis."

GRAPES. Grapes are the perfect finger food to lovingly feed to one another. Thought to be the oldest fruit in the world, grapes have also been considered aphrodisiacs for nearly as long. They contain very healthy flavonoids that act as antioxidants within your body. Nothing makes you feel more catered to than when your partner hand-feeds you grapes like you are a member of the royalty.

MANGOS. Mangos are exotic, flavorful, and juicy. The mango is an extremely healthy fruit, loaded with vitamins A and C. It is ideal for dieting because its high fiber content makes it filling. It also works as a gentle laxative or diuretic.

ORANGES. This yummy fruit has served as an aphrodisiac in China, and as a holiday treat in many cultures. Oranges are loaded with vitamin C. In fact, over 100 percent of the recommended daily allowance of vitamin C is contained in a single orange. Oranges provide other benefits, including important amounts of potassium, calcium, magnesium, and phosphorus. Anthocyanins, which give blood oranges their red hue, may be helpful in preventing some cancers. All varieties of oranges boast a significant amount of fiber, vitamin A, and folate. They also have only about seventy calories each.

PASSION FRUIT. Of course, passion fruit on this passion-filled diet is a natural.

PEACHES. The peach has a seductive shape. The crease in the fruit resembles the lips of a woman's vagina. Peaches also contain vitamins and minerals that contribute to your health and well-being.

PEARS. Pears are a very appropriate fruit for a diet in which you are working as a pair! Again, this fruit has a lovely, phallic shape and is filled with minerals. Very low in calories and sodium and full of fiber, pears are a great supplement to a weight loss diet. The pear also contains a lot of potassium that is critical, together with calcium, to the process of bone formation. It is also important for the proper regulation of liquids in the body and for the well-being of the nervous system.

PINEAPPLES. Rich in vitamin C, pineapples are used in homeopathic treatment for impotence. Add a pineapple spear to an occasional sweet rum drink for a tasty prelude to an evening of passion.

WATERMELON. Watermelon is one of the lycopene leaders among fresh fruit and vegetables. A plant pigment found in only a few red plant foods such as tomatoes and watermelon, lycopene is thought to have powerful antioxidant capabilities and may help to prevent certain diseases.

Meat

Don't be afraid to eat meat on the Ultimate Sex Diet; just take care not to treat your lover like a piece of meat. If you do not eat any meat, you can end up with zinc and protein deficiencies, which can lead to reduced libido and low sperm counts according to Sheldon Saul Hendler, M.D., Ph.D., an assistant clinical professor of medicine at the University of California, San Diego. On this diet, we recommend eating limited portions of lean red meat one to two times a week, and skinless chicken and fish on the remaining days. Fish, shellfish (we will elaborate on oysters as aphrodisiacs below), and red meat are especially high in zinc. If you are a vegetarian, you will need to eat fruits and vegetables that provide the nutrients found in meats and fish. For example, you can supplement your diet with pine nuts, which are rich in zinc. They've been stimulating libidos since medieval times.

Meat is also helpful to nutrition in other ways. According to Elizabeth Ward, R.D., a Boston-based nutrition consultant, "[t]he protein in the meat will naturally boost levels of dopamine and norepinephrine, two chemicals in the brain that heighten sensitivity during sex." Of course, it is a good idea to check with your physician or nutritionist to determine how much meat is right for you.

Seafood

Fish are an important part of any healthy diet. They provide the protein that your heart needs, and are lower in fat than meat. While you can enjoy most fish, the Environmental Protection Agency and the U.S. Food and Drug Administration recommended in March 2004 that young children and women who are pregnant or may become pregnant, not eat shark, swordfish, king mackerel, or tilefish because they contain high levels of potentially harmful mercury.

OYSTERS. Oysters are very sensual foods that are widely known as romantic delicacies. They were even regarded as aphrodisiacs by the Romans in the second century A.D. Their sexual powers may be due to the belief that the oyster resembles the "female" genitals. Besides their benefits as an aphrodisiac, oysters are also good sources of protein. Of course, as with other seafoods, you should be aware of the potential for them to be infused with overly high concentrations of harmful chemicals. So always check the news for any advisories about the safety of fish being caught in your region.

SALMON. Salmon is a powerhouse of nutrition. It is a good source of protein and is packed with omega-3 fatty acids, which are powerful antioxidants. Omega-3 fatty acids may also aid in raising serotonin levels in the brain, lift moods, and lower feelings of irritability. As an added benefit, salmon contains fish oils that may help lower cholesterol levels. Other oily fish, such as sardines and herring, could also be part of your diet. All are rich in vitamins A, B, and D, and also phosphorous and calcium, which are well-known libido boosters.

Spices and Herbs

Add some spice to your life! Herbs and spices add flavor to your food, and they might also jazz up your love life. Basil, garlic, ginger, ginseng, pepper, clove, and the other herbs and spices mentioned below will make your meals tastier and more satiating.

GARLIC. The heat in garlic supposedly fires the flames of passion. Unless you freshen your breath after eating this healthy delicacy, your love life will flame out.

GINGER. Ginger root in any form is a stimulant to the circulatory system. Plus, don't forget Ginger from *Gilligan's Island*; she was quite a beauty! I used to aspire to be her.

GINKGO BILOBA. Reportedly, this plant optimizes sexual pleasure by easing muscle tension and increasing blood flow to the brain and sexual organs.

GINSENG. Ginseng is reputedly a means of boosting libidos!

LICORICE. The Chinese have used licorice for medicinal purposes since ancient times. Chewing on bits of licorice root is said to enhance sexual desire and has also been known to work as an appetite suppressant. Try a cup of calorie-free, licorice-flavored herbal tea as an afternoon treat.

MUSTARD. Mustard is said to increase the libido. Add some mustard to your salad, or make a delicious Dijon sauce to pour over your chicken, steak, or vegetables.

ONIONS. Onions not only add flavor to your meals; they also stimulate blood flow. Arab folklore claims that an aphrodisiac drink of onion juice mixed with honey was the original Viagra. Take care to keep a toothbrush and minty Tic-Tacs handy when you pack your meals with our ring-shaped friends.

VANILLA. The scent and flavor of vanilla is believed to increase lust. Add a teaspoon to any food, including coffee or tea. Some of the new diet vanilla sodas are so delicious, they taste like dessert and have zero calories! However, you need to limit your consumption of diet sodas due to health concerns.

WASABI AND HORSERADISH. Wasabi and horseradish speed up the body's metabolism and are believed to be effective aphrodisiacs for increasing sexual performance.

Nuts

Nuts are great! No, not just husbands and boyfriends! The ones you buy in the store.

Nuts are high in fiber and in "good" fat, and are a great source of protein. Eating nuts may lower the risk of heart disease, stroke, diabetes, and dementia. They are also a wonderful source of vitamin E. Eating nuts can satisfy your hunger, although the amount consumed needs to be closely watched because nuts contain an abundance of calories. When you eat nuts, watch the serving size and eat no more than 200 calories' worth. I particularly enjoy the following nuts:

ALMONDS. Almonds have been symbols of fertility throughout the ages. Their aroma is thought to induce passion in females.

BRAZIL NUTS. Brazil nuts are a great source of selenium, which is a trace mineral that helps keep sperm cells healthy. These nuts are also a good source of vitamin E, an antioxidant that helps protect the body from damage by free radicals, according to Keith Ayoob, R.D., a spokesman for the American Dietetic Association.

GINKGO NUTS. These are quite popular and improve blood circulation to the extremities of the body, also boosting libido.

PISTACHIOS. Pistachios are great nuts to eat if you are in the mood for snacking. The fact that you need to de-shell each one slows the eating process, and the nuts themselves are quite small, so you are less likely to consume an overabundance of calories. Buy the unsalted variety.

WALNUTS. Walnuts were used by the Romans in fertility rites, and they are believed to increase libido.

Grains

Despite what some low-carb diet advocates claim, whole grains are a nutritious and important part of any healthy diet. Eat grains like oats as part of your breakfast, and experience the effect by bedtime! Oats are believed to increase the release of testosterone in both males and females and thereby boost libido.

CEREAL AND WHOLE-GRAIN BREADS. The right non-sugary breakfast cereals can be quite healthy. Choose whole-grain brands loaded with thiamin and riboflavin. Both vitamins help you use energy efficiently, so you stay more alert throughout the day. Fortified whole-grain breads and cereals are also high in niacin, a vitamin that's essential for healthy skin, nerves, and the digestive tract. It also helps to lower the levels of "bad" cholesterol within the body. Finally, choose whole grains that are high in fiber so that you will stay full longer, and maintain your regularity.

Dairy Products

CHEESE. "Cheese is one of the best foods you can eat for your teeth," says Mathew Messina, D.D.S., a spokesman for the American Dental Association. "It's a good source of calcium to keep your teeth strong. [Moreover], eating cheese can lower the levels of bacteria in your mouth and keep your teeth clean and cavity free." Due to their high fat content, limit your intake of cheeses and focus on the low-fat varieties. For example, low-fat cottage cheese is quite flavorful and satisfying.

MILK. The calcium in milk helps strengthen bones so you and your partner can make love more vigorously. Milk also provides many other essential nutrients needed to keep the body healthy. Drink the low-fat varieties.

YOGURT. Yogurt is an excellent source of protein, calcium, riboflavin, vitamin B-12, and a host of beneficial live bacteria, which many healthcare professionals believe helps maintain intestinal health and provide relief from certain vaginal infections. The active cultures in yogurt may also boost the immune system.

Other Foods and Drinks

CHAMPAGNE. The celebratory carbonated "drink of love" gets many of us in the mood. Again, take care to drink in moderation. As Shakespeare wrote in Macbeth, alcohol "provokes the desire, but it takes away the performance."

COFFEE. According to some, coffee drinkers reportedly are more sexually active than non-coffee drinkers. How can we test this theory in our own homes?!

EGGS. Eggs are a good source of B vitamins, which are extremely beneficial nutrients that may help you relax and increase your sexual desire.

SOY AND TOFU. Soy and tofu (which is made of soybeans) are wonderful sources of protein. Soybeans are also a source of plant estrogrens that may help relieve PMS. Tofu also been reported to help fight certain types of cancers and reduce cholesterol. Though plain tofu can be very bland, there are several ways it can be prepared to make it more palatable. Among my favorites are grilled, barbecued, or marinated tofu.

SUGAR-FREE COCOA. This is a frothy treat, good for satisfying chocolate cravings without much of the fat or calories. Cocoa may also help keep arteries flowing freely. Penny Kris-Etherton, a professor of nutrition at Pennsylvania State University, also indicated that it is a good source of the flavonoids thought to retard the buildup of harmful cholesterol.

SUGAR-FREE FUDGE POPS. Just like sugar-free popsicles, fudge pops are low in calories and fun to play with. Best of all, they can be used to satisfy chocolate cravings.

SUGAR-FREE JELL-O. This dessert is great for satisfying sweet cravings, yet is extremely low in calories and fun to play with, especially when you adorn your lover with it. Add fat-free whipped cream for extra flavor and pleasurable entertainment.

SUGAR-FREE POPSICLES. Very low in calories, they can satisfy sweet cravings and can be very seductive when eaten slowly while staring at your partner. Of course, they can be used for extra fun in the bedroom.

TEA. Soothing and delicious, tea helps promote peace of mind on a stressful day. Also, tea is quite healthy. According to John Weisburger, a Ph.D. researcher at the American Health Foundation who has performed several studies on the subject, tea reduces the risks of cancer and heart disease. It also strengthens the bones of postmenopausal women. Weisburger cites research indicating that tea's antioxidants may be ten times more effective than vitamin C and twenty-five times more potent than vitamin E in neutralizing harmful free radicals in the body.

WATER. The benefits of drinking "nature's wine" cannot be underestimated. For most people, drinking ample amounts of water during the day speeds the body's chemical processes, enhances energy production, and improves the appearance of the skin. The first symptom of dehydration is fatigue. Drink as much water as possible throughout the day to stay energized, healthy-looking, and more appealing to the one you love. Think of the difference between a grape and a raisin. Which do you find more visually appealing?

WINE. A glass or two of wine can add romance and atmosphere to any afternoon or evening. Wine relaxes us and helps to stimulate our senses. Red wines also contain flavonoids, which act as cancer-preventing antioxidants and may reduce the levels of "bad" cholesterol in the body. However, be sure to limit your wine intake because excessive alcohol consumption can lead to a night of slumber rather than sexual adventure.

Aphrodisiac Indulgences

Ahhhh . . . What pleasure! However, the following are indulgences and should be eaten in moderation.

CHOCOLATE. Chocolate is infused with chemicals thought to affect neurotransmitters in the brain related to our feelings of pleasure and satiety. It also contains theobromine, a mild stimulant with a mood enhancing effect. Dark chocolate is a rich source of flavonoids, which can reduce the damaging effects of "bad" cholesterol. It contains more antioxidants (cancer-preventing substances) than red wine. One secret for arousing passion is to combine these two potent aphrodisiacs. Try a glass of Cabernet with a bit of dark chocolate for a sensuous treat on special nights.

FROZEN YOGURT. Similar to regular yogurt, though not quite as healthy, low-fat frozen yogurt contains high levels of calcium and phosphorus, two minerals that strengthen your bones and add to your muscles' energy reserves. They also boost your libido! In addition, all that calcium can make your orgasms more powerful, since the muscles that control ejaculation need calcium in order to spasm and contract properly, according to Sara Brewer, M.B., author of *Increase Your Sex Drive*. Eating machine-made frozen yogurt may be an even healthier way to consume this treat. The machine infuses the dessert with air, so the serving seems larger although it actually contains fewer calories than the variety available in the hard-packed cartons.

TRUFFLES. These exquisite rare treats were one of the Romans' favorite aphrodisiacs. The appeal is undoubtedly in the rich feel that truffles produce in your mouth. Their musky aroma is said to stimulate and sensitize the skin to touch.

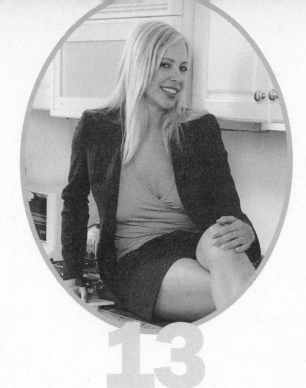

13

THE 2-WEEK SEX DIET

On this diet, the terms are simple. We select from each of the recommended food groups to ensure that the intake during the day is well-balanced and nutritional. Calorie counting is a headache and can take the joy out of a meal. Instead, we have a few simple rules to help keep you in the ballpark but won't have you obsessing over that extra five calories in a piece of gum. Besides, your partner will surely attest that fresh breath is definitely worth the indulgence!

The general rule of thumb is that a serving-sized portion for many of the food groups is considered the size of your fist . . . I guess that makes it a rule of fist. Also, in the first two weeks, no late night snacking is allowed. Any time you have the urge, replace it with activity with your partner. You also must engage in sexual activity (preferably using the recommended positions) at least five times a week. I recommended three to five times during the work week, and twice per day on the weekends. The rules for this program includes four to five (or more) fistfuls of fruits and colorful and flavorfully prepared vegetables, three to four grains, two dairy, and two proteins per day.

In the first two weeks, the only alcohol allowed is wine or

champagne—you may have one glass on three separate nights if you wish. After two weeks, you may cut out one dairy and instead incorporate one indulgence a day that is approximately 200 calories and has no more than fifteen grams of fat.

Finally, the only fat-free foods should be yogurt (which is still yummy), sour cream, and skim milk. One percent fat milk is acceptable as well. This is simply because many fat-free foods lack flavor and are a waste of calories in my opinion. Fat-free cheese tastes like plastic. Cream based salad dressings tend to taste a bit off as well. Stick to low-fat, low-sugar, low-calorie dressings (like vinaigrettes), and make sure you keep the serving to no more than one or two tablespoons each time.

Fat-free bread is just silly! Bread has very little fat, it's the starch and white flour consumption that is not conducive to dieting. Even on the few days when you do allow yourself some whole grain bread, don't worry about the fat. Also, do not eat any so-called "carbohydrate-free foods" where it is clearly unnatural for the foods to be in this state. Carb-free bread, pasta, yogurt, and ice cream are just strange. I've sampled them and they all seem to have odd consistencies and they taste terrible. One last note, vegetarians, please feel free to substitute any meats included on the plan with the vegetarian versions of the foods. I actually am a big fan of soy "deli meats", "to-furkey", and Boca anything.

Just to recap before we get into the daily plan, here's the quick and dirty rule list:

1. Rule of Fist

2. No late night snacking unless it is on your partner

3. Sex at least five times during the week

4. Daily food group selection: four to five (or more) fistfuls of fruits and vegetables, three to four grains, two dairy, two proteins

5. Alcohol is only one wine or champagne per day, allowed three times per week

6. Skip fat-free foods (except for those mentioned above)

7. No carb-free foods where it seems unnatural for them to be in this form

8. After the first two weeks, one starch can be swapped for one alcohol

The 2-Week Sex Diet plan was created with the collaboration of Toby Amidor. Toby Amidor, M.S., R.D., is a registered dietitian who earned her master's degree in clinical nutrition and dietetics from New York University. She attended NYU with her mother (yes, they were in the same classes) and even graduated at the same time. For the past seven years, she has been an instructor at The Art Institute of New York City where she teaches potential chefs about nutrition and food safety. She was published in *The All New Joy of Cooking* (under "Know Your Ingredients"), where she helped compile the food composition table of more than three hundred foods. Toby also consults for various food marketing and food safety companies and media outlets including television, Internet, newspapers, and magazines.

Day 1:

Drink water throughout the day and with meals. (Flavored sparkling waters can also be substituted.)

Breakfast:

A high-fiber cereal, such as Kashi, that has a nice flavor and contains a minimum of 5 grams of fiber. Mix in berries, and eat it with vanilla soy milk for extra flavor (low-fat versions are available).

Coffee or tea (Drink something with a nice flavor, or perhaps add a flavored cream.)

Mid-Morning Snack:

Flavorful fruit, such as a peach, mango, or star fruit.

Lunch:

Chef salad with ham, turkey, 1 tablespoon bacon bits, 1 tablespoon shredded cheese, 1 tablespoon low-fat dijon dressing. Sugar-free Jell-O made or topped with apple slices, water, or flavored sparkling water.

Mid-Afternoon Snack:

Herbal tea, bag of flavored soy crisps (they're quite good, actually; I like the white cheddar flavor) and baby carrots.

Dinner:

Broccoli and cauliflower (2 fistfuls) with melted low-fat cheese (1 oz.), poached salmon with a store-bought low-fat lemon dill sauce (fist-sized portion).

Dessert:

Fistful of cherries and whipped cream on your partner.

Day 2:

Drink water throughout the day and with meals. (Flavored sparkling waters can also be substituted.)

Breakfast:
Coffee or tea (Drink something with a nice flavor, or perhaps add a flavored cream.)
Tomatoes with basil and a dash of olive oil, 2 hard-boiled eggs flavored to taste (I like pepper and a dash of Tabasco sauce), sliced cantaloupe.

Mid-Morning Snack:
Small bag of celery or carrots, flavored to taste (low-fat dressing, salt, mustard, etc.).

Lunch:
Side salad with only dark-green vegetables and low-fat dressing. Sandwich on whole grain bread, turkey lunch meat, mustard, or low-fat mayo.

Mid-Afternoon Snack:
Small container of cottage cheese topped with peaches, diet drink of choice.

Dinner:
Side salad of lettuce, cucumber, and tomato with 1 tablespoon low-fat vinaigrette, baked chicken cooked in low-fat, low-sodium mushroom soup, sauteed spinach with garlic, and 1 teaspoon of olive oil.

Dessert:

Baked apple with cinnamon and nutmeg, squirt of whipped cream on top. Optional: Glass of wine.

Day 3:

Drink water throughout the day and with meals. (Flavored sparkling waters can also be substituted.)

Breakfast:
Coffee or tea (Drink something with a nice flavor, or perhaps add a flavored cream.)
Cottage cheese with berries, mixed with a serving of high-fiber cereal.

Mid-Morning Snack:
Handful of pecans and almonds mixed
Sugar-free cocoa made with skim milk

Lunch:
Tuna salad with low-fat mayo, relish, and lettuce
2 clementines or 1 medium orange
String cheese or Dannon 70-calories Light and Fit smoothie

Dinner:
Side salad of lettuce, tomato, and cucumber with 1 tablespoon of low-fat vinaigrette.
Small portion (fistful) of lean filet mignon, cooked winter squash, steamed broccoli with a touch of olive oil and garlic.

Dessert:
Sugar-free Popsicle or Pudding Pop.

Day 4:

Drink water throughout the day and with meals. (Flavored sparkling waters can also be substituted.)

Breakfast:
Coffee or tea (Drink something with a nice flavor, or perhaps add a flavored cream.)
Low-fat or nonfat yogurt with berries, Boca meatless sausage

Mid-Morning Snack:
Lunch meat rolled in one 6" tortilla with mustard and horse radish.

Lunch:
Grilled chicken Caesar salad with low-fat dressing, or ask for the dressing on the side and take your 1–2 tablespoons.
15 grapes

Afternoon Snack:
Carrots, broccoli, and yellow squash with hummus, 3 tablespoons

Dinner:
Japanese Theme Night:
20 edamame
Miso soup
Sushi, minimize the rice and replace with cucumbers

Some restaurants have brown rice sushi available or you can use brown rice if you make it yourself.

Dessert:
Sliced pineapple
Optional: Glass of saki

Day 5:

Drink water throughout the day and with meals. (Flavored sparkling waters can also be substituted.)

Breakfast:
Coffee or tea (Drink something with a nice flavor, or perhaps add a flavored cream.)
Quaker instant oatmeal made with 1 tablespoon of cashews and blueberries, and topped with cinnamon, V-8 (NOT THE SPLASH!) or make your own fresh vegetable juice.
Honeydew melon.

Mid-Morning Snack:
Small serving of cheese and low-fat turkey pepperoni on 3–4 whole wheat crackers.

Lunch:
Egg salad with low-fat mayo on lettuce stuffed in a whole wheat pita. Sliced red and green peppers.
Orange

Mid-Afternoon Snack:
Strawberries with powdered sugar.

Dinner:
Korean Theme Night:
Kimchee
Clear soup
Korean barbecue beef wrapped in lettuce

Dessert:
Poached pear topped with cinnamon and a drizzle of chocolate syrup

Day 6:

Drink water throughout the day and with meals. (Flavored sparkling waters can also be substituted.)

Breakfast:
Coffee or tea (Drink something with a nice flavor, or perhaps add a flavored cream.)
Two-egg omelette (egg white or egg-beaters for the truly dedicated), with low-fat mozzarella cheese, peppers, mushrooms, and green onions

Mid-Morning Snack:
Ham and American cheese roll, fistful of baby carrots with mustard or low-fat mayo

Lunch:
Side salad of lettuce, tomato, and cucumber with 1 tablespoon of low-fat vinaigrette. Two low-fat turkey hot dogs and mustard in a whole wheat pita or whole wheat bun.

Afternoon Snack:
Cup of chocolate soy milk and 4 strawberries

Dinner:
Mexican Theme Night:
Gazpacho soup
Fajita: Grilled steak, shrimp, onion, peppers, spice, served with dollop of fat-free sour cream. Slice green peppers and celery, and dip in salsa.

Dessert:
½ mango
Optional: Make your own sangria with a glass of white wine, mixed with club soda, and chopped fruit.

Day 7:

Drink water throughout the day and with meals (flavored sparkling waters can also be substituted).

Breakfast:
Coffee or tea (Drink something with a nice flavor, or perhaps add a flavored cream.)

Boca meatless sausage, 2 poached egg whites, 1 slice whole grain toast with a teaspoon of all fruit (no added sugar) jelly or jam.

Mid-Morning Snack:
Fat-free/low-calorie yogurt with kiwi slices.

Lunch:
Vegetarian chili or low-fat turkey chili (made with kidney beans, chilli powder, tomatoes, and onions).

Mid-Afternoon Snack:
Low-fat cheese stick with 15 grapes

Dinner:
American Barbecue Theme Night (choose two of the meat dishes given below):
Steak kabob made with green and red bell peppers and onions.
No-bun–grilled chicken with low-sugar barbecue sauce.
No-bun burger: Try lean ground beef, turkey, tofu, or veggie burger (I prefer the Boca Burger brand) with lettuce, tomatoes, pickles, mustard, and a dollop of low-fat mayo.

Dessert:
1–2 dark chocolate squares and ½ medium banana (the darker the chocolate the better).

Day 8:

Drink water throughout the day and with meals. (Flavored sparkling waters can also be substituted.)

Breakfast:
Coffee or tea (Drink something with a nice flavor, or perhaps add a flavored cream.)
Smoothie made with sugar-free nonfat yogurt, milk, 1–2 fistfuls of equally combined strawberries, blueberries, and raspberries.

Mid-Morning Snack:
Trail mix (total should be a handful eaten): pecans, cashews, almonds, dried raisins, dried cranberries

Lunch:
Tuna nicoise salad with 1 slice of 100 percent whole wheat bread

Mid-Afternoon Snack:
Fistful of fruit salad made with apples, pears, grapefruit, and pineapples, topped with a teaspoon of vanilla and cinnamon.

Dinner:
Chinese Food Theme Night:
Spinach soup
Steamed chicken and shrimp with broccoli (add soy sauce or low-sugar teriyaki sauce), or
Steamed pork and green beans (mix with a ginger sauce)
Fistful of brown rice

Dessert:
Fortune cookie (it's a small indulgence, but it's low in calories), for extra fun, buy the X-rated fortune cookies and surprise your partner.

Day 9:

Drink water throughout the day and with meals (flavored sparkling waters can also be substituted).

Breakfast:
Coffee or tea (Drink something with a nice flavor, or perhaps add a flavored cream.)
Four egg white omelet filled with spinach and goat cheese. One slice of whole grain bread on the side, topped with a sugar-free jam. Sliced cantaloupe on the side.

Mid-Morning Snack:
Turkey jerky with sliced veggies (carrots, celery, and broccoli).

Lunch:
Caesar salad with grilled chicken, carrot soup (with no cream in the base).

Mid-Afternoon Snack:
Luna bar.

Dinner:

Italian Theme Night (choose one chicken dish below):

Tomato and mozzarella salad with basil

Chicken marsala: Make your own with chicken, mushrooms, and mushroom soup

Chicken scaloppine-sautee chicken breast in 1 tablespoon butter, 1 tablespoon olive oil, chicken broth, lemon juice, and salt

Asparagus, boiled, then pour mixture of lemon juice, dijon mustard, and olive oil to top

Side: A fistful of whole wheat pasta

Dessert:

3 strawberries and ½ sliced kiwi with whipped cream

Optional: Wine

Day 10:

Drink water throughout the day and with meals. (Flavored sparkling waters can also be substituted.)

Breakfast:

Coffee or tea (Drink something with a nice flavor, or perhaps add a flavored cream.)

Low-fat deviled eggs (You can replace the egg filling with a tofu eggless salad if desired and top with cayenne pepper.)

Grapefruit sliced in half, sprinkled with Equal

Mid-Morning Snack:

Fiber-rich crackers with Laughing Cow cheese

Lunch:
Minestrone soup, Greek salad with low-calorie dressing

Mid-Afternoon Snack:
Zucchini, celery, and broccoli with low-fat dressing

Dinner:
Seafood Night:
Caesar salad
Shrimp or seafood cocktail
Steamed oysters
Artichoke with 1 teaspoon olive oil and garlic flavoring

Dessert:
Fat-free chocolate mousse pop
Optional: Wine

Day 11:

Drink water throughout the day and with meals. (Flavored sparkling waters can also be substituted.)

Breakfast:
Coffee or tea (Drink something with a nice flavor, or perhaps add a flavored cream.)
Smoked salmon rolled with low-fat cream cheese and capers

Mid-Morning Snack:
Sliced apple sprinkled with cinnamon and nutmeg

Lunch:
Oriental chicken salad (salad, chicken, mandarin oranges, slivered almonds, low-fat, low-calorie dressing)
1 slice of whole grain bread

Mid-Afternoon Snack:
Bag of soy crips and 1 cup of herbal tea

Dinner:
Side salad of lettuce, cucumbers, tomato, and a tablespoon of low-fat vinaigrette
Orange roughy fish with ginger
Creamed spinach or green bean casserole (Green beans baked in low-fat, low-sodium cream of mushroom soup; please check soup ingredients that cream was not added. Serve with crushed onion flavored soy crisps sprinkled on top for added crunchiness.)

Dessert:
Sugar-free Jell-O with orange sliced inside
Optional: Glass of champagne

Day 12:

Drink water throughout the day and with meals. (Flavored sparkling waters can also be substituted.)

Breakfast:
Coffee or tea (Drink something with a nice flavor, or perhaps add a flavored cream.)

Melon fruit salad (made with honeydew, watermelon, and cantaloupe. I like to add star fruit for presentation.)
Three-egg white omelet with slices of turkey bacon and mushrooms mixed in.

Mid-Morning Snack:
Cheese slices with cherry tomatoes and carrot sticks

Lunch:
Steamed calamari salad
4 strawberries

Mid-Afternoon Snack:
Broccoli, cauliflower, red pepper slices, and hummus

Dinner:
Pork chops: Bake with onion soup and add a no-sugar-added applesauce with cinnamon and nutmeg.
5 mini new potatoes with skin, halved and baked with a touch of olive oil and pepper.
Broiled tomatoes with 1–2 tablespoons parmesan cheese

Dessert:
8–10 frozen grapes and 1–2 square (1-ounce) of dark chocolate

Day 13:

Drink water throughout the day and with meals. (Flavored sparkling waters can also be substituted.)

Breakfast:

Coffee or tea (Drink something with a nice flavor, or perhaps add a flavored cream.)

Chocolate banana smoothie made with sugar-free chocolate mousse Popsicle, ½ packet sugar-free cocoa, skim milk, Equal, ice, and a banana.

Mid-Morning Snack:

Trail mix (total should be a handful eaten): pecans, cashews, almonds, dried raisins, dried cranberries

Lunch:

A Subway-brand Atkins-friendly sandwich, such as the turkey breast and bacon melt, or the chicken and bacon ranch sandwiches or any 6 Under 6 sandwich. You can also have any sandwich made with Atkins-friendly bread.

Mid-Afternoon Snack:

Peach

Dinner:

Polish Theme Night:

Beet soup with hard-boiled egg sliced in half.

Side salad with lettuce, cucumbers, tomato, and 1 tablespoon of low-fat vinaigrette

Grilled low-fat kielbasa (only one serving) with mustard and beet relish, served with cabbage or stuffed cabbage with lean ground beef in tomato juice.

Dessert:

Lime sugar-free Jell-O made with cottage cheese and pineapple

Day 14:

Drink water throughout the day and with meals. (Flavored sparkling waters can also be substituted.)

Breakfast:
Coffee or tea (Drink something with a nice flavor, or perhaps add a flavored cream.)
Oatmeal with raisins and cinnamon and topped with skim milk

Mid-Morning Snack:
Veggies (carrots, green and yellow peppers, and celery sticks) dipped in salsa

Lunch:
Strawberry pecan spinach salad with raspberry vinaigrette

Mid-Afternoon Snack:
Nonfat yogurt topped with 1 tablespoon of granola

Dinner:
Fistful of lentil soup
Turkey meatloaf with no breading, made with onions, and flavored to taste
Side of string beans topped with 1 teaspoon of olive oil and garlic
Mixed berries drizzled with sugar-free chocolate syrup (preferably on your partner).

As mentioned earlier, after the first two weeks, you should continue to stick to the general diet plan, but you can now substitute one snack for a 200-calorie indulgence each day. I recommend treats like low-fat frozen yogurt topped with fresh fruit slices and low-fat brownies, but everyone has their own tastes. You can also substitute a low-carb beer, or a drink with hard liquor for the dairy as well. Maintain this program until you reach your ideal weight. Depending how much you need to lose, it should take most people about two months to achieve this goal. Vary the meals in the preceding pages as you wish, but stick to the general foods and rules of the diet plan. NO CHEATING!!!! Especially in the first two weeks. This is the most crucial time.

14

FIGHTING CRAVINGS:
DON'T CRAVE SWEETS,
CRAVE YOUR SWEETIE

The problem is most of the things that are good for us—exercise,
salads and early nights—are pretty boring. So it's good to hear that
something fun, like sex, actually has masses of health benefits.

—Christine Morgan, *London Mirror,* February 12, 2004

Have you ever had the feeling that you would "simply die" if you did not indulge in something sweet, greasy, or fattening immediately? Do you often find yourself sitting in front of a television set mindlessly chomping away, only to realize that you have consumed an entire bag of Doritos? We all go through points in the day where our hunger for unhealthy foods can feel overwhelming. What we need to learn is which snacks minimize caloric intake but maximize the eating experience. That knowledge, and a little will power, will help you avoid unhealthy bingeing.

The first step is to take a moment to analyze the feeling of hunger when it arrives. Are you really hungry, or are you just bored and looking for something to fill the void? Of course, you can sometimes wonder about your urge to have sex in these terms, but at least making love doesn't expand your waistline! Are there particular times during the day when you

> We all go through points in the day where our hunger for unhealthy foods can feel overwhelming. What we need to learn is which snacks minimize caloric intake but maximize the eating experience. That knowledge, and a little will power, will help you avoid unhealthy bingeing.

feel the urge to snack? I have observed that environment plays a major part in my own snacking habits. If I buy a box of candy from a newsstand I pass on my way home from work, when I pass that newsstand again the next day I may crave candy even if I am not hungry. When this happens, I make a concerted effort to change my routine. For example, I leave work by a different route, until I don't associate passing a certain location with eating.

Once a bad influence or a negative eating pattern is identified, it is necessary to prepare for it. A great strategy is to turn your thoughts to having sex. When you are feeling the need for something sweet in your life, think instead about your first, or most erotic, sexual experience with your partner. Think about when you are going to have sex with your partner again. Imagine a creative new twist to your lovemaking that will add a magical new touch to the experience. You can even follow the "Sex Duet" rule and call your partner to have a little "sex talk."

I have found this technique to be particularly effective in the late afternoon or early evening when I am on my way home from work. I am always incredibly hungry at that time of day, and since I have a one-hour commute home, there is a great deal of downtime which could be spent (horror of horrors!) snacking. If I am not careful, I can accidentally end up eating enough Oreos and Milk Duds to fill a small truck. I have discovered that if I focus on looking forward to seeing Ben, and I think about what I am going to do to him in bed that night, it becomes hard to think about anything else. Incidentally, we have found that a fantastic time to make love is immediately when we both get home from work. If we have been stressed out or annoyed that day, it is a great way to push those negative thoughts out of our minds and also get in some stimulating exercise. This helps us avoid the risk of getting so tired that we choose an early bedtime over a romp in the sheets.

Of course, personal schedules and meal times are major factors that influence when people have food and sex cravings, so work out the best strategy with your partner. Try to accommodate each other's "moments of extreme need" or MEN (who seem to have them fairly frequently).

Now, I understand that sometimes the hunger pains are real and that you actually do need to eat something rather than just attempting to distract yourself. You should then try munching slowly on a snack rich in fiber rather than grabbing any "empty calorie wonders." Basically, begin most snacks or meals with a vegetable or two. Celery or green peppers are wonderful starters. You can sprinkle each with a little salt or dip them into a low-fat dressing to create a satisfying snack. Fruits are also great because their rich flavors and fibers can really quench your hunger. If you are in the mood for a more substantial snack, try sticking to foods that take longer to eat. String cheese or low-fat cottage cheese with a few pieces of fruit should do the trick.

> Try to accommodate each other's "moments of extreme need" or MEN (who seem to have them fairly frequently).

If you absolutely cannot resist chips at a party or cookies at work, control your intake. Eat just a few chips and make a commitment that you will not return for seconds. Grab a small handful of chips and dip, or one or two cookies, and sit down to eat. Unlimited quantities of readily available sugary or fattening snacks are your worst enemy. Do not bring them into your home, and avoid them outside the house.

Another strategy is to buy packages of food that contain

individually wrapped treats, so the portion is set for you. If you cannot resist ice cream or ices, stick to the low-calorie varieties such as sugar-free pops and low-fat ice cream, or buy the packages that come with individual cups of ice cream. When you have to give in to something that has limited nutritional content, at least you will eat an individual serving and no more. If you are dying for pizza, occasionally allow yourself to eat a slice of the Lean Cuisine or Healthy Choice frozen pizzas. Make them into a meal, not a snack. These pizzas are lower in calories and fat than the greasy slices sold at the corner.

Whatever snack you choose, be sure to pay attention to its nutritional content. Always read the nutritional information on the package. Try not to eat any snack that exceeds 200 calories per portion or one that has a fat content above ten grams.

Also be aware of how much you are enjoying a snack as you eat it. How does it taste? Is it adequately providing the taste you were craving? Do not wait until you have gorged on an entire package of snack food to realize that it was not what you were craving in the first place. If you take a couple of bites and realize that you are not really enjoying the snack, do not waste the calorie intake it entails. Just stop eating it. If there is even a remote chance that you will end up eating what you are craving anyway, it is pointless to eat another snack that you do not enjoy. On the other hand, if you are craving a specific taste, substitute a healthier version of the snack. For example, substitute soy crisps for potato chips or a low-calorie chocolate fudge Popsicle for a piece of chocolate

> Remember to plan for snack attacks, and do your best to replace your passion for unhealthy foods with passion for your partner.

cake. Also, despite what you may think, eating something healthy does not cancel out eating something fatty. Just because you eat an apple first, it does not mean the Bill of Rights gives you the freedom to eat a piece of cheesecake!

Be smart about what you do choose to eat. There are some so-called nutritional bars on the market that are packed with calories and taste terrible. Substitute more natural, fresher foods for these outrageously expensive "health" bars.

Remember to plan for snack attacks, and do your best to replace your passion for unhealthy foods with passion for your partner. Try recalling the most romantic thing your partner has done for you, or plan to do something naughty or nice for him or her. The goal is to get the giddy feeling in your stomach that was there at the start of the relationship. Nothing is a better appetite suppressant than that good old lovesick puppy feeling. Not even seven facials a week will produce the glow that comes from a wonderful sexual encounter. There are very few problems that a good orgasm cannot cure, or at least make you forget. It starts in your mind, and the longer the anticipation, the more fulfilling the experience will be.

Foods to Avoid

We recommend completely avoiding the foods listed below during the first two weeks of the Ultimate Sex Diet, and severely limiting them thereafter. However, I realize that we all have our weak moments, so I will suggest some substitutes to fill your cravings, yet keep you in line so you do not regain the weight you have already lost.

BEER. Stick to very limited quantities of light, low-carb beers.

CAKE. If you absolutely must eat cake, try a slice of moist angel food cake. It is relatively low in calories and fat. Angel food cake is especially delicious with a few berries or fruit slices on top.

CANDY. If necessary, suck on hard candies because they take longer to finish. If you must eat an unhealthy type of candy, such as gummy bears or a candy bar, try freezing the candy so it takes longer to eat. Jelly beans have relatively few calories per bean. Make sure to separate the portion you will eat and put away the rest of the bag.

CHIPS. Instead of high-fat corn or potato chips, try soy crisps. If you really "need" potato chips, try the baked versions. Stick to a small, snack-size bag of the chips or count them out before you eat them. Better yet, have a bag of reduced-calorie, no-salt (or lightly salted) popcorn. Half a bag of these treats has less than 200 calories.

COOKIES. Try the low-fat versions instead. Set aside one or two and eat them very slowly.

CORN. Try corn on the cob. It is fun to eat and the portion is easier to control.

FRIED FOODS. Try baked foods sprinkled lightly with bread crumbs instead of eating fried foods. Grilled foods can be just as tasty.

FRUIT JUICES. These generally contain too much sugar. Try one of the "light," low-calorie versions of the juices. Even better, eat the fruits themselves. Their fiber will help satiate your hunger.

HARD ALCOHOL. Have a small glass, but do not drink it with tonic, which is usually high in sugar. Try mixing it with diet soda, club soda, lime juice, or other low-calorie beverages. Stick to very limited quantities of wine and champagne when the mood is right for love.

ICE CREAM. Low-fat versions are almost as tasty. Frozen yogurt is an excellent substitute. As discussed above, the soft-serve version of frozen yogurt (or, if you must, of light ice cream) can save you calories because the air pumped into them makes each serving seem bigger.

PIE. Try to eat only the filling. If you bake the fruit yourself, it can taste like pie filling, with less sugar and fat. I enjoy baked apples sprinkled with cinnamon and nutmeg. A baked, whole-wheat pita pocket can be substituted if you must have the pie filling wrapped in something crust-like.

PIZZA. Try a Lean Cuisine or Healthy Choice frozen pizza. They are fairly tasty and far less fatty than the greasy slices you get at the pizza parlor.

POTATOES. Limit your intake of potatoes. Try sweet potatoes. When prepared well, they can be quite delicious. They are also are high in fiber. Try not to add butter or other unhealthy toppings to your potatoes. Eat the baked varieties instead of those that are fried.

SUGAR. Use very small quantities or natural substitutes.

WHITE PROCESSED BREAD. Stick to limited portions of whole-grain breads. If you must have a piece of white bread, have a slice of light, low-calorie bread.

WHITE SEMOLINA PASTA. Avoid high-calorie, cheesy pasta dishes and substitute modest portions of whole-wheat pasta with freshly-made tomato sauce instead. Or have a frozen diet TV dinner such as Healthy Choice or Lean Cuisine, which have controlled portions.

WHITE OR INSTANT RICE. Substitute brown rice instead and control your portion.

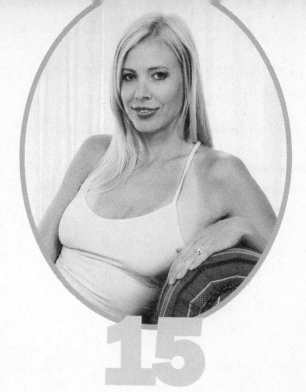

15

COMPARING THE DIETS

People should avoid popular low-carb and low-fat diets that can produce initial weight loss but rarely work in the long term. Study after study shows that more moderate restrictions are more likely to last permanently.

—Katherine Tallmadge, American Dietetic Association,
The Associated Press, June 2, 2004

We all know there are countless diet programs available today. The options range from numerous fad diets and crash diets, to low-fat and low-carb diets. Which is best? Let's examine a few of the programs and compare them to the Ultimate Sex Diet.

One does not need to review all of the scientific literature on nutrition to realize that the real secret to lasting weight loss is simply to eat healthy foods, reduce your caloric intake, and exercise regularly. This is the strategy that the Ultimate Sex Diet makes so simple and pleasurable. The wonderful advantage of the Ultimate Sex Diet is that even if you do not have the time or desire to go to the gym, you can still get plenty of exercise at home, particularly in bed! You're encouraged to regularly do simple exercises that will tone and strengthen key parts of your body so that you will be healthier and more attractive to your partner. On the Ultimate Sex Diet, you are not

One does not need to review all of the scientific literature on nutrition to realize that the real secret to lasting weight loss is simply to eat healthy foods, reduce your caloric intake, and exercise regularly. This is the strategy that the Ultimate Sex Diet makes so simple and pleasurable.

forbidden to eat foods from any particular food groups. Instead, you are encouraged to eat moderate amounts of lean protein, fruits and vegetables, low-fat milk and dairy products, and even carbohydrates (particularly from whole grains and nuts). With the goal of limiting your portions to sizes that will satisfy your hunger and meet your nutritional needs, we have discussed how to eat your foods slowly while savoring each bite. On the Ultimate Sex Diet, you are encouraged to get all of the nutrition and love that you need. Moreover, no other diet program comes with a built-in, live-in, support network like this one! I highly doubt that any other program will result in lovemaking as wonderful as the Ultimate Sex Diet. Vive la difference!

> I highly doubt that any other program will result in lovemaking as wonderful as the Ultimate Sex Diet. Vive la difference!

LOW-CARB DIETS. The first diet approach we will discuss is the low-carb obsession that has recently spread so rapidly across America. The low-carb regimen has even spread to soda and candy manufacturers, who are tripping over themselves to create low-carb versions of their products. The problem is that many of these low-carb foods are actually not healthy for you; in fact, they can be high in calories. In my opinion, these processed "low-carb foods" defeat the purpose of why these diets were ever allegedly successful in the first place.

One of the reasons the low-carb diets first became popular was that they were an easy way to limit snacking. When the low-carb mania first began, there were few low-carb sweets to fill the void between meals. If you were craving a cookie, you were left hungry or you were snacking on healthy foods, such as moderate amounts of raw vegetables and nuts. Now, with the flood of low-carb cookies and other snacks, people on low-carb diets can eat "low-carb" food all day, but still snack, overeat, and not lose weight. The scientific reason why the low-carb diets were supposed to work was that the reduction in carbohydrates would force the body to burn fat for energy. However, this won't happen when you consume large quantities of high-calorie, low-carb foods.

Even before the availability of a huge number of low-carb foods, the low-carb diets were problematic in many ways. When people participated in a strict low-carb diet regimen and consumed virtually nothing but proteins, their bodies were deprived of essential vitamins and nutrients for the duration of the program. This is not healthy, even temporarily. Moreover, even if dieters do lose weight initially on low-carb diets, once they return to their normal lifestyles and eating habits, their weight loss is usually quickly reversed and they gain back all, or nearly all, of the weight they lost.

In a Reuters report published June 22, 2004, a coalition of health experts argued that "popular low-calorie diets are leading Americans to poor health and are spawning a rip-off industry of 'carb-friendly' products."

THE ATKINS DIET. This is a diet program that drastically reduces the amount of carbohydrates in one's diet. Many people love it because when they first begin the diet, they can eat all the high-fat steak, bacon, and cheese they want. Does that sound healthy to you? I don't think so. Many nutrition and health experts share my view. Consuming fat may lead to increased risk of cancer, heart

> I have kept my excess weight off for over three years while on a very healthy regimen of sensible eating and amazing lovemaking—the Ultimate Sex Diet!

disease, and other chronic illnesses. In contrast, I have kept my excess weight off for over three years while on a very healthy regimen of sensible eating and amazing lovemaking—the Ultimate Sex Diet! I am still slim and happy, and I have a great sex life!

THE SOUTH BEACH DIET. This is a modified low-carb diet, similar to Atkins, but it limits the permitted intake of fatty foods and allows more vegetables. From what I understand, many participants get sick at the sight of Laughing Cow Cheese halfway through the program because of its frequent presence in the plan. More seriously, the absence of fruit and high-fiber whole grains in the first two weeks of the program and the still very high amount of fat permitted on this diet are major concerns. Most importantly, the South Beach Diet does not include a lot more sex in its program like the Ultimate Sex Diet does. It sounds like it might get very lonely on that deserted beach!

On June 23, 2004, a large group of doctors, scientists, and nutritionists announced the formation of the Partnership for Essential Nutrition. to warn that low-carb diets such as the Atkins and South Beach regimens were leading Americans to poorer health and creating a misleading industry of "carb-friendly" products. Jeff Prince of the American Institute for Cancer Research, a member of the new Partnership, stated that "eating vegetables, fruits, whole grain and beans, which are all predominantly carbohydrates, is linked to a reduced risk of cancers, heart disease, stroke, diabetes and a range of other chronic diseases." He warned that those who follow diets focused on high fat and animal protein consumption are "increasing the risk of developing cancer, heart disease, stroke, type-2 diabetes and other ailments."

LOW-FAT DIETS. Low-fat diets also present challenges and concerns. Because low-fat foods have been popular for decades, there are countless choices available for virtually every food you could possibly desire. Therefore, there is no guarantee that your caloric intake will be limited on these diets, and eating thousands of empty carbohydrate calories can pack on the pounds. Additionally, some low-fat versions of foods do not accomplish the goal of satiating cravings. People on low-fat diets often feel entitled to eat larger portions if they know a food is lower in fat, which defeats the whole purpose of the diet! The focus should be on the nutritional value of the foods you are consuming and not solely on the amount of fat in them. Eating five pounds of gummy bears, which are virtually fat-free, does not mean you are getting any healthier. Many people who engage in low-fat diets also have a tendency to neglect the appropriate consumption of healthy fibers. High-fiber foods are important for keeping the body's digestive system cleansed and healthy. A recent study published in the Journal of the American Medical Association suggested that high-fiber cereals and other whole grains may even aid in the prevention of certain cancers.

Many people on low-fat diets consume unhealthy amounts of foods

> Eating five pounds of Gummi bears, which are virtually fat-free, does not mean you are getting any healthier.

> Many scientific studies have highlighted the importance of the critically important nutrients, proteins, and vitamins found in the lean meats, fish, and nuts that may be in short supply on some low-fat diets.

containing sugars and processed white flour. Some also avoid fish and nuts because of the significant fat content in these foods.

> Most of the time, people who try fad diets starve themselves for a few days and then end up bingeing and weighing even more than they did before they started riding the fad diet roller coaster.

This approach is very unhealthy because fish and nuts are filled with "good fats," which have enormous health benefits. Moreover, fish and nuts contain omega-3 fatty acids, which have been shown to reduce the risk of heart disease and may even fight Alzheimer's disease. Many scientific studies have highlighted the importance of the critically important nutrients, proteins, and vitamins found in the lean meats, fish, and nuts that may be in short supply on some low-fat diets.

FAD DIETS. Most fad diets are among the least successful of diet programs. If you are thinking about participating in one, save yourself the time, money, and effort. Most of the time, people who try fad diets starve themselves for a few days and then end up bingeing, and weighing even more than they did before they started riding the Fad Diet Roller Coaster. The ups and downs of these roller-coaster rides are simply not as much fun

> Weight loss that occurs gradually and represents a more pleasurable lifestyle is healthier for your body and is more likely to achieve the lasting results you want.

as those at amusement parks. This is why the Ultimate Sex Diet is better. The ups and downs on the sex diet actually result in very pleasant body sensations. Many of the names of fad diets out there, such as the cabbage soup diet and the grapefruit diet, simply make me laugh. Who would actually want to do one of these diets knowing that the pounds will almost surely return right away? In my opinion, it's a waste of time, and often money, to participate in a program that does not have a realistic chance of becoming a permanent source of healthy weight loss. As the saying goes, no one ever became fat in one day, and no one ever became skinny in one day. Avoid diets that promise you unrealistic immediate weight loss. Weight loss that occurs gradually and represents a more pleasurable lifestyle is healthier for your body and is more likely to achieve the lasting results you want.

16

SEXUAL HEALING: THE AMAZING HEALTH BENEFITS OF SEX

A good sexual relationship is essential to good health.

—Dr. Barbara Bartlick, Professor of Psychiatry

Founder, Human Sexuality Programs

Weill Cornell Medical College, New York

Knight Ridder Newspapers, February 13, 2004

Of course you will love losing weight with a more intensive love life, a healthier diet, and the slimming exercises we've discussed earlier. But are you ready for even better news? The Ultimate Sex Diet can also help you live a healthier, longer life by having sex more often! Isn't that the best news you've heard all day?!

In fact, there are new scientific discoveries every year on the health benefits of sex. No, it's not because there are a large number of lusty scientists out there itching for any excuse to get someone in bed with them! It is because researchers are increasingly focusing on the enormous medical benefits of staying active between the sheets. Though most of us do not need much convincing to want more sex, it is important that we understand how more loving each day keeps poor health at bay.

When one is aroused, more of the hormone oxytocin is secreted into the body, which causes the release of endorphins. The increased oxytocin levels may not only lead to orgasm, but,

Of course you will love losing weight with a more intensive love life, a healthier diet, and the slimming exercises we've discussed earlier. But are you ready for even better news?

according to some studies, may also provide pain relief. That's because the natural opiates released during sex, such as endorphins and corticosteroids, act as painkillers and relieve many sources of aches and pain within the body, from headaches to minor arthritis. This is why couples often sleep better after making love. Additionally, measurements performed at the Masters and Johnson Institute have shown that the uterine contractions brought about by orgasm (triggered by oxytocin) are just as powerful as those that occur during the labor preceding childbirth. Women can use these orgasmic contractions and relaxations of the uterine muscles that occur during sex to relieve the cramps caused by PMS.

> Though most of us do not need much convincing to want more sex, it is important that we understand how more loving each day keeps poor health at bay.

It is no surprise that arousal leads to increased blood flow to all bodily organs, including the brain. As the fresh blood supply is delivered throughout the body, your cells, organs, and muscles are saturated with fresh oxygen and hormones. As the used blood is removed, you also remove waste products from your body that may cause fatigue and even illness.

Sex, like other physical exercise, increases the body's production of testosterone, the hormone that helps regulate sexual activity, according to Dr. Karen Donahey, the director of the Sex and Marital Therapy Program at Northwestern University Medical Center. The testosterone boost from sex is good for men and, surprisingly, for women as well. It not only boosts libido, but also strengthens the bones and muscles. Funny that more sex equals the production of more testosterone, which leads to a

> The natural opiates released during sex, such as endorphins and corticosteroids, act as painkillers and relieve many sources of aches and pain within the body.

desire to have more sex, which leads to the production of more testosterone.

The hormone DHEA promotes sexual excitement and then increases in response to arousal. Dr. Theresa Crenshaw, author of *The Alchemy of Love and Lust*, says DHEA may be the most powerful chemical in our personal world. It may help to balance the immune system, improve cognition, promote bone growth, and maintain and repair tissues, keeping your skin healthy and supple. It may also contribute to cardiovascular health and even function as an antidepressant. According to a Sun Media report dated February 24, 2004, men having frequent sex cut their risk of having heart attacks and strokes in half.

> The testosterone boost from sex is good for men and, surprisingly, for women as well. It not only boosts libido, but also strengthens the bones and muscles.

As we've discussed earlier, regular sex is a great form of moderate exercise, and its dividends include the many benefits that moderate exercise provides: it strengthens the heart, lowers body weight, increases stamina, and improves cholesterol levels. In fact, it even helps tip the HDL/LDL (good/bad) cholesterol balance toward the healthier HDL side. Moreover, a Pennsylvania study indicated that people who have sex at least once a week boost their body's immunoglobulin A, an antibody known to boost the immune system, by 30 percent. According to the Mayo Clinic, moderate aerobic exercise also stimulates the growth of tiny blood vessels in your muscles. Since these capillaries help your body to deliver more oxygen to your muscles and remove wastes such as lactic acid,

> Men who have sex at least three times each week may have a decreased risk of developing prostate problems.

they can lessen chronic muscle pain, including chronic back pain.

Men who have sex at least three times each week may have a decreased risk of developing prostate problems. This finding is supported by a study that CNN discussed on April 7, 2004. The study involved almost 30,000 health professionals, ranging in age from forty-six to eighty-one, who were surveyed on the frequency of their ejaculations during various stages of their lives. During the approximately eight years of follow-up to the study, 1,449 men developed prostate cancer. Findings from the study showed that groups categorized as having the two highest activity levels (thirteen to twenty ejaculations a month and at least twenty-one ejaculations per month) were linked with decreased prostate cancer risks of 14 percent and 33 percent, respectively. One theory for this is that frequent ejaculations help flush out cancer-causing chemicals or reduce the development of calcifications that have been linked with prostate cancer. Additionally, ABC News reported on December 5, 2003, that research showed a causal relationship between infrequency of ejaculation and cancer of the prostate. To produce seminal fluid, the prostate and the seminal sacs take zinc, citric acid, and potassium from the blood and concentrate them up to 600 times. The same effect may happen when these organs concentrate carcinogens, which is why it is better to flush them out through ejaculation.

> Making sex more frequent and intense may keep your brain sharp for years to come. That means you'll be able to remember those exciting lovemaking sessions more vividly!

According to Denise Foley, author of *As Good As It Gets,* sex may also improve your memory and make you smarter. Studies show that intense stimulation, such as that which occurs during sex, can produce chemicals in the brain that trigger the formation of new dendrites, the filaments attached to nerve cells that allow neurons to communicate with one another. Lawrence Katz, a professor of neurobiology at Duke University, has stated that the more dendrites you have, the better you learn and the more you remember. So, making sex more frequent and intense may keep your brain sharp for years to come. That means you'll be able to remember those exciting lovemaking sessions more vividly!

As I mentioned at the outset of the book, an active sex life may also help us age better and live longer. Dr. David Weeks, a clinical neuropsychologist at Scotland's Royal Edinburgh Hospital, conducted a study of 3,500 people ranging in age from eighteen to one hundred two. In his book, *Secrets of the Superyoung*, Dr. Weeks

> An active sex life may also help us age better and live longer.

concluded that sex sharply slows the aging process. Additionally, a British study of 1,000 men found that those who had at least two orgasms a week had half the death rate of their countrymen who indulged in sex less than once a month.

In fact, scientists are also constantly finding new and unusual benefits from sexual activity. In May 2001, *Men's Health* magazine carried one interesting suggestion: "When you get the hiccups, don't breathe into a paper bag. Have sex. A forty-year-old Israeli man with chronic hiccups tried everything to stop the annoyance. . . . Then his doctor suggested he try intercourse. The hiccups stopped right after he ejaculated—and they haven't been back for a year."

> WOW! Sex reduces stress and pain, strengthens your heart and muscles, reduces your risk of heart disease and cancer, and even helps you live longer. This is "Dr. Kerry" telling you to get into bed and call me (to thank me) in the morning.

WOW! Sex reduces stress and pain, strengthens your heart and muscles, reduces your risk of heart disease and cancer, and even helps you live longer. This is "Dr. Kerry" telling you to get into bed and call me (to thank me) in the morning.

17

EMBRACING YOUR
NEW LIFESTYLE

The more sex, the happier the person.

—David G. Blanchflower, Dartmouth University

and Andrew Oswald, Warwick University

Money, Sex and Happiness: An Empirical Study

National Bureau of Economic Research, May, 2004

When you think about it, we are all walking testaments to the miracle of sex. Two wonderful people made love, and, with God's help, made each of us! Therefore, when we participate in the Ultimate Sex Diet we are giving tribute to the human reproductive system and to the process by which we were created. Okay, so today there are sperm banks and in vitro fertilization. However, if you are reading this book now, that is not how you were created! I know it's a bit difficult to envision our parents in this light, but it's the truth!

Now let's make sure we remember the steps necessary to successfully participate in all areas of this sexy diet regimen. First, we are going to discuss with our partners the wonderful benefits of going on the Ultimate Sex Diet, and gently convince them to participate in the diet with us. We are going to keep track of our food intake and exercise more frequently. We will document, through notes and photographs, the incredible body changes and weight loss we will experience on the diet. We will become more sensual, sensitive beings, and make efforts to improve our appearance,

When you think about it, we are all walking testaments to the miracle of sex.

grooming, and eating habits. We will maintain a positive opinion of ourselves and our partners and embrace the intimacy and positive feelings we achieve with them.

Make love more often, more passionately, more creatively, and more intensely.

For the first two weeks, we will avoid all foods on the Do Not Eat list. After the first two weeks, we will continue to eat leaner, smarter, and healthier. We will control our portions, and focus on the healthy foods and aphrodisiacs we've discussed instead of on eating unhealthy indulgences or fattening snacks.

We will spend time on activities, such as walking, biking, and hiking that we enjoy doing alone or with our partners. Moreover, we will regularly do the warm-up, teasing, and toning sexercises to improve our bodies and our love lives.

Most importantly, we will make love more often, more passionately, more creatively, and more intensely.

NEVER STOP LOVING

Sex . . . is the activity that produces the largest amount of happiness.

— Daniel Kahneman, "Measuring the Quality of Experience,"
Working Paper, 2003, Princeton University

I t is very hard to believe, but it's over already! You barely felt a thing! Oh, I am sure you felt many wonderful sensations in bed. However, the diet was relatively painless, wasn't it? After all the waiting and time spent anticipating, I'm sure the experience was virtually painless. Who would have guessed that after all the talk, the operation would be so simple.

No, we're not talking about the sex (at least I hope not)! We're talking about the successful weight loss and body transformation that has occurred since you began the Ultimate Sex Diet. You undoubtedly have a glorious glow about you and an added bounce in your step. Now that you have completed the Ultimate Sex Diet you should feel energized, confident, and satisfied—without the usual deprivation, depression, and frustrations of the other diets you've tried. I hope you enjoyed the diet program as much as I did. To be honest, I still enjoy the Ultimate Sex Diet very much and hope I will always be on it!

The exercise portion of this program should not end just because you have achieved your goal weight.

If you have reached your ideal weight, congratulations! How about a celebratory lovemaking session? That's right, the exercise portion of this program should not end just because you have achieved your weight goal. Now that you have rediscovered and reenergized your passion and feelings for your partner, don't start neglecting them again. You are a new person now, and you should never stop having a terrific sex life. Life is short, so enjoy the ride, especially the free one that your partner gives you! Always shower your partner with compliments, love, and affection. Don't close the newly opened channels of communication, and continue loving your body, loving yourself, and loving each other. Never forget that a positive frame of mind is the first step to success at love and at life.

> Life is short, so enjoy the ride, especially the free one that your partner gives you! Always shower your partner with compliments, love, and affection. Never forget that a positive frame of mind is the first step to success at love and at life.

I hope this book has taught you that the wonderful, sensual feelings that lovemaking creates throughout your body should become an important, frequent, and permanent part of your life. In their research survey, "Money, Sex and Happiness: An Empirical Study," economists David Blanchflower and Andrew Oswald concluded that "the more sex, the happier the person." Now you can testify to the truth of their findings.

Please pass on the secret to everyone you know. You may be met with skepticism, but anyone who knows you well will have witnessed the change that has occurred to your body and to your outlook on life. Let everyone know about the powerful secret and success of the Ultimate Sex Diet.

> Let everyone know about the powerful secret and success of the Ultimate Sex Diet.

May we always cherish our partners and appreciate everything they have done for us. When all is said and done, it is wonderful to have someone who can lift up our spirits when we are at our most vulnerable, and mend our state of mind when it is not filled with confidence and hope. Our partners see us naked and love our bodies. They are the only ones who have fully witnessed the extraordinary body transformation we have undergone on this diet. They should always be treated with the love, affection, and respect that they need and deserve.

Cheers to us, the successful participants on the Ultimate Sex Diet! May we live long, healthy, happy, and satisfying lives, filled with the pleasure and power of love.

The book has ended, but with the right effort, your amazing sex life will go on and on. Enjoy!

AFTERTHOUGHTS . . .

Share Your Success with the Ultimate Sex Diet . . .

Why not inspire others?

If the Ultimate Sex Diet has helped you or someone you love slim down, lose weight, or build a more passionate relationship, please let me know. Send your inspiring comments (up to 250 words) to kerry@truecouragepress.com. Before and after photos, if available, would also be appreciated. Your encouraging words my help hundred of thousands of men and women to lead healthier and happier lives.

Thank you,
Kerry

ULTIMATE LOVING—FREE.

Are you interested in the latest news and breaking stories on:

- Health and Fitness
- Love and Relationships
- Sex and Sexual Health

Do you want expert advice on your most critical questions about health, fitness, self, love, and relationships?

Do you want a supportive community to help you lose weight and gain a more passionate relationship?

Then sign on—free—to
WWW.ULTIMATELOVING.COM

The free information you need. The discounts and free gift you'll treasure.